LIVING DAILY WITH DEMENTIA:
'IT WASN'T ME'

Living Daily with Dementia: 'It Wasn't Me'

by

Shirley Ashman

~

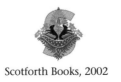

Scotforth Books, 2002

First published in 2002 on behalf of the author by
Scotforth Books,
Carnegie House,
Chatsworth Road,
Lancaster LA1 4SL,
England
Tel: +44(0)1524 840111
Fax: +44(0)1524 840222
email: carnegie@provider.co.uk
Publishing and book sales: www.carnegiepub.co.uk
Book production: www.wooof.net

British Library Cataloguing-in-Publication data
A catalogue record for this book is available from the British Library

ISBN 1-904244-03-3

Typeset by George Wishart & Associates, Whitley Bay
Printed and bound in the UK by Antony Rowe Ltd, Chippenham

Dedication

This book is dedicated to:

Olwen, my late mother, whose memory I honour, and George my father – without him this book would not have been written.

Alwyn, my husband, whose support and encouragement has been invaluable – especially providing me with endless cups of tea whilst in the process of writing!

Matthew and Michael, my sons who were always ready to give an extra hug of comfort when needed. (Remember your promise, boys!)

Contents

Acknowledgements

I would like to thank everyone who helped me to bring this book into being. They include three people who, unknown to them, were the source of confirmation from God that I should put pen to paper. These are Wendy Banwell (my Pastor's wife), Sarah Tummey and Ken Withers (friends of Bethlehem Baptist Church, Thomastown).

Then there were the manuscript readers/correctors/advisors – Joyce Harris and David Roberts whose help and counsel were greatly appreciated.

Thanks must also go to the staff of the Community Services Department, National Health Trust, Day Care Unit, Carers Association, Alzheimer's Disease Society and the Residential Home. Please note that other than family members' names, all original names of people and establishments have been changed in order to maintain confidentiality.

Above all, I would like to express my thanks and praise to God who enabled me to tell my story and bring about something positive and creative out of what otherwise would seem to be such a negative situation.

Foreword

The book that you hold in your hands is a true story. It tells, in part, the story of an illness that over the last ten years seems to have dropped out of the sky onto society, and become commonplace affecting huge numbers of families. Shirley, in her diary, clearly portrays the physical and mental pressures of caring for, and trying to arrange the best possible help and treatment for her Dad. But there is a spiritual side to this story that seems to bring light and hope into the situation. Shirley's faith has helped her enormously in coming to terms with an illness that many can relate to. Jesus says in the Gospel of Matthew, 'Come unto me, all you who are weary and burdened and I will give you rest' (*Matthew 11:28*) and to know that in itself – what a comfort it can be.

Shirley has grown up with the scriptures and came to an understanding of who Jesus was and what He had done for her on the Cross at the young age of twelve. Through many trials and struggles over the past forty-eight years of her life, Shirley has grabbed onto the many wonderful promises the Bible clearly gives, which have enabled her to have the strength to put pen to paper in the hope that others may be helped. I know that there were many tears shed during the writing of this diary as we both prayed together. However, these were not all tears of sorrow, there have also been tears of joy as she has clearly experienced the Lord moving and controlling many of the events during this stressful time.

As a pastor, my heart goes out to those who find themselves in a similar situation, because this illness is often more traumatic for the carer than for the patient. But as Shirley clearly shows in her story,

God made a way when there seemed to be no light at the end of a long tunnel. 'Hear my prayer, O Lord; listen to my cry for mercy. In the day of my trouble I will call to you, for you will answer me' (*Psalm 86:6-7*).

I pray that this book may be a practical help and a source of comfort to those who, through no fault of their own, find themselves in a similar situation. If you have never found the reality of God in your own life, and therefore tried to convince yourself that He simply did not exist, after reading this book it will become clear that God is real. And I pray that you will discover the scarlet thread that runs through every page holding it all together – Jesus Himself.

Reverend E. Banwell BA

Introduction

'I just can't seem to see the light at the end of the tunnel.' 'I'm so alone.' 'No-one understands what I'm going through.' If you have found yourself either thinking or saying these sentiments, then this book was written with you in view! There is no magic formula or recipe to follow in order to bring about a change to the situation – just a faith in Someone Who has the power to change lives and attitudes. My prayer is, that after reading the following story, your life will never be the same again.

God bless you.

CHAPTER 1

The Telephone Call

9 August 1999 My cousin Ken rang at 11pm and said that he and his wife Gaynor had been out for the evening, and that whilst they were walking home, they saw Dad at the bus stop waiting to go home. Of course there were no buses at that time of night and Ken had been drinking and would definitely not entertain the thought of driving. Unfortunately, John (Ken's brother) was also unavailable and so Ken rang me. When I eventually arrived at Aunty Joyce's, Gaynor explained that Dad had come up to visit at 8.30pm thinking it was the morning and he was totally unaware of the right time. This was despite the fact that it was getting dark – no amount of explanation would convince Dad. However, in the end I managed to drive him home and settle him down and I told him that the next day, when he woke up it would be Tuesday and it would be the morning. I came home and cried my heart out.

10 August 1999 I rang Derek (my only brother who lives in Leicester) to advise him on what had happened last night. I told him that I would like to take Dad to the doctor but that I was unsure as to how Dad would react. I suggested that maybe the doctor could come out to see Dad at his flat, but I was so ashamed of anyone visiting because of the state of the place. Since Mam died, he has just let himself and the flat go and there is nothing he will let me do to help – it's so very difficult! Derek suggested that I get the flat cleaned up and then call the doctor in. After phoning Derek, I rang Dad to see how he was and he appeared to be as right as rain! There was no apparent sign of confusion and I was somewhat relieved   but not entirely satisfied. On calling on Dad this evening, he said that he was having trouble with his telephone and so I rang BT to report the fault.

1 September 1999 I rang Dad to let him know that whilst sorting through some paperwork I had found two fully paid-up insurance policies and on enquiring, it was found that Dad could surrender them for a cash sum if required. He was so relieved because he confessed that he was 'worried sick'. He'd had letters from the Council to say that he was in arrears with his rent and also that his Council Tax payments were in arrears. Another letter had come from the Water Rates Authority saying the same thing. What has happened to my Dad? He said that the insurance money would come in very handy at the moment. On further investigation, I found out that his rent had not been paid since the 7th June and also it was at this time that the Council Tax and Water Rates had stopped being paid! Perhaps the anniversary of Mam's birthday had upset him?

I also discovered a problem with junk mail and it has caused problems with Dad financially. His bank account, which at one time had £3,000.00 three years ago, now only had £7.00 in it! He had been sending money away to various companies at UK addresses and also abroad. In my opinion, they are all 'cons' and 'scams' and I tried to explain to Dad but he became aggressive and wouldn't listen to reason.

3 September 1999 The redemption forms to claim Dad's insurance came through the post and I had a photocopy of Mam's death certificate and asked Dad to sign the documents before posting them off. Dad seemed very relieved that I was sorting things out for him and he vowed that he would never send any more money away again! He promised me faithfully because he could see how upset I was over the issue. Alwyn and I left Dad's flat hoping that, at last, he was beginning to see sense.

CHAPTER 2

The Sort Out

6 September 1999 We popped in to see how Dad was and to give him a method of sorting out his pension on a weekly basis in order to be able to pay off his arrears more quickly. He went into an aggressive mood and said he wanted to pay off his debts 'in one go and not in dribs and drabs' and that he was going to continue to try and win a fortune by sending off money to these competitions etc. I said that wasn't the answer and reminded him of his promise to us that if he should get any more junk mail he wouldn't open it but put it in the bin or the fire. Dad became very agitated when I took the letters etc and said that I was going to burn them. He told me, 'Do what the hell you like!' It was at this point of sheer exasperation and disappointment that I snapped back at Dad, 'No, Dad – you do what the hell you like – I'm not interested in your problems any more – get your act together on your own!' Alwyn and I walked out of Dad's flat in a very dismissive way, leaving Dad to ponder these things in his own company! Our next visit to him was to be on Friday.

10 September 1999 This visit was our first communication since our 'walk-out' on Monday and the atmosphere was decidedly cool! I explained to Dad that his welfare was our concern and that I was going to write to the House of Commons via our MP to ask if the Government could do anything about the practice of these conmen as quite a number of people we knew had also been receiving such nuisance mail. I apologized for my outburst on Monday and explained that I loved him and was only interested in his well-being, and I was so upset that he was making his situation worse by still replying to these letters. He apologized too and said, 'I won't do it again, Shirl, I can see how it's upsetting everyone – including me – and so I've finished with that now. I promise you faithfully.' I heaved a huge sigh of relief – at last we seemed to be getting through!

13 September 1999 Dad wrote a letter to the Council saying that a standing order was not required from his bank account but that he would be paying his rent by cash every week. (I had explained by telephone and also in writing to the Rent Officer that Dad was about to receive a sum of cash from an insurance policy that had long since matured and that the full amount of arrears would then be settled from the proceeds).

22 September 1999 Alwyn and I went to the Council Office and paid Dad's rent arrears. We called back to Dad's and gave him the receipt. I then sorted out every receipt that I could find with regard to each of his outgoings. A file was made out for RENT, COUNCIL TAX and WATER RATES. Dad was in such a muddle previously but now that he accepted my help he seemed relieved that some order was now beginning to emerge out of the chaos!

CHAPTER 3

The Storm

1 October 1999 Alwyn and I called at our usual time – 6.30pm. Dad was out. It was raining heavily and the signs were that he hadn't long gone out (the kettle and teapot were still warm, the toaster had been used and there was jam on the knife – Dad had just had his 'breakfast' so he thought). I immediately rang Aunty Joyce who told me that Dad had visited her earlier in the day and he left about 2pm. I then rang to see if Dad was at his friend's house (Geraint lives in the next street) but he wasn't there. I went down to the next block of flats where Mrs Williams lives (the ninety year old lady who calls in to see Dad every day) but he wasn't there either. By this time, I was both praying and panicking! Gaynor (Ken's wife) rang to ask if Dad had come back and I broke down in tears at this point and said, 'No!' As Ken is a policeman and would know what to do with regard to initiating a search, Gaynor asked me to ring her back at 9pm if Dad hadn't returned. At this point, the whole of the housing estate was plunged into darkness due to the electricity power-cut in the storm. Then my prayers were answered! Here came Dad, stumbling through the garden gate. I was standing on the doorstep and went rushing to fetch him in from the torrential rain. What a sorry state he was in! I broke my heart and asked him if he was alright and where had he been. He said he went shopping and was waiting for a bus and then he realized it must be the wrong time as there were no buses forthcoming and it was getting dark. He was soaking wet and freezing cold and whilst he was changing into dry clothes the electricity came back on line. Alwyn and I made him a hot cup of tea and drew up the fire. I told Dad I was going to contact the doctor but he became annoyed and refused point-blank. I said that it was because I loved him and that we were concerned for him that I just had to make an appointment. He reluctantly agreed and we left him in a much better situation than when he came in!

2 October 1999 I phoned Dad's GP and the earliest appointment we could have was for 10.40am on Monday, 4th October. I rang Dad to advise him of the time and date and asked him to make a note of the appointment on his calendar. On asking him how he was feeling today, he replied that he was alright and didn't know what all the fuss was about!

4 October 1999 Dad and I arrived at the surgery and I explained my concerns regarding Dad's uncharacteristic behaviour – his confusion over the time of day, his general forgetfulness over paying his bills etc. As Dad also suffers from recurring varicose vein trouble in his left leg which causes him considerable discomfort from time to time, I brought this matter to the doctor's attention. The doctor noted from his records that Dad hadn't received a 'flu or pneumonia injection and so after advising Dad to rub on the cream he'd prescribed for his leg problem, he asked Dad if he wanted to have these two vaccinations. Dad replied that he would but he had previously told me that he would never have another 'flu jab ever again as it had made him ill the last time. (He later told me that he didn't like to say 'No thank you' to the doctor!).

The doctor prescribed some tablets for Dad and advised me that he would refer Dad to a special clinic for an assessment and asked me if I would be able to take him if an appointment was made. I said, 'Of course' and so we left the surgery and were asked to make an appointment to see the doctor in a month's time.

19 November 1999 Dad's second appointment with his GP (a little later than a month's time due to the fact that Alwyn and I moved house on 22nd October). Dad was still complaining of his leg pain and the doctor, after examining Dad's leg, said that there was nothing else that he could do except refer him to the hospital for an operation to remove the varicose veins. However, this was not advisable due to Dad's age. When Dad had pain, he was told to take pain-killing tablets as and when required. The matter regarding Dad's confusion was being referred to a doctor in Ysbyty Cwm Rhondda (Rhondda Valley Hospital) and we would be receiving a letter in due course.

CHAPTER 4

Conspiracy

3 December 1999 Arrangements have been made for a doctor from Ysbyty Cwm Rhondda to visit Dad at home today with a view to making an initial assessment of Dad's condition. Various questions were asked by the doctor who made it quite clear to Dad that he must not look to me for any clues to the answers. A mental arithmetic test was also carried out. After a while, Dad agreed to allowing me to do his washing – this indeed was progress! Following the completion of the assessment, I accompanied the doctor to the garden gate whilst Dad made a cup of tea. It did appear from this initial interview that the diagnosis is likely to be that Dad is in the early stages of a form of dementia. However, the doctor advised that Dad would have to have blood tests taken and a special X-Ray Scan of his brain. An appointment would be made shortly. I thanked the doctor for being so frank with me and prayed to the Lord for strength to bear whatever was in store for us as a family in the future.

6 December 1999 Dad at bus stop in Porth at 11.45pm. No buses arrived but a van driver pulled up and gave Dad a lift to Ystrad (Aunty Joyce's). Ken brought him home and phoned me to explain what had happened. He also said that on two separate occasions, Dad had asked Gaynor to count his money as he didn't know or couldn't work out how much loose change he had. I shared with Ken what had taken place with the specialist doctor and in view of the recent events we were both concerned as to Dad's safety. Anyone could have picked him up at that late hour and mugged him or worse – left him for dead. I said I would bring the matter to the doctor's attention. However, the doctor would not be available until Wednesday morning.

8 December 1999 Alwyn and I had to be over Abercynon this morning by 9am as it was the day for our grandson's School Concert. However, I rang the doctor in the interval to explain what had developed with Dad since last Friday. The doctor said that he would ask the CPN (Community Psychiatric Nurse) to call in to see Dad.

17 December 1999 Bethan Rees (CPN) visited Dad at 11am and together we filled in a Question and Answer Form. This basic information which we provided helps Bethan to monitor Dad. Her approach was very caring and professional and she put my mind at ease to know that at least we were not alone in this situation.

27 December 1999 Gaynor rang at 12.30pm to say that Dad had upset Aunty Joyce over the phone. He was convinced that she had been in the flat and he was talking to her. Aunty Joyce was supposed to have left suddenly without saying where she was going. Gaynor explained that Aunty Joyce had never left her home, but Dad became very cross when Gaynor tried to advise him of this fact. She suggested Dad should let both myself and the doctor know what he had experienced as the doctor would be able to give him the appropriate help that he needed. I waited for Dad to ring me, but when he didn't, I rang Bethan's extension. However, I was unable to speak to her and so left my name and number asking for her to ring me when she was available. Alwyn and I went up to see Dad and asked him if he was alright. I said that Gaynor had rung me and I was very concerned as she said that Dad was upset. Dad then became convinced that Gaynor and Aunty Joyce were 'working it between them'. I asked Dad what he meant by that and he accused them of 'making up tales between them to tell the doctor and to show him that I was going mad'. I tried to reassure Dad that this wasn't the case at all and that both Gaynor and Aunty Joyce thought too much of him to do anything like that. I also explained that he didn't have a brain clot as he had already told Gaynor, and once again I went through what the doctor had said about the necessity of a brain scan and blood tests and tried to reassure him that he wasn't going mad. What he'd experienced was probably a very vivid dream. He seemed to be calm and accepted what I said and then we left, telling him that we would call the next day as usual at 6.30pm.

28 December 1999 I rang Bethan's number but was told that no-one would be in until tomorrow due to the Christmas and Bank Holiday period. Alwyn and I called to see Dad as usual at 6.30pm and were greeted with, 'You're early!' Dad thought it was the morning and said that he'd just got up and lit the fire. There was a plate of sandwiches on the table and I asked Dad about them. He said he'd made them for Aunty Joyce but she left them saying she wasn't hungry and then she left. I made a cup of tea and noticed that Dad was still pondering over something and then he asked, 'What day is it?' I replied that it was Tuesday evening, not morning and he intimated that his memory was failing him again. I suggested that we play cards (as is our usual custom and practice) to try to get Dad's mind focusing on something that we always did together at a certain time during our visit. This was followed by watching TV. The programme 'Eastenders' was on and Dad said, 'I thought that this programme was on in the evening – what's it doing on this time of the morning?' I reassured him again that it was the evening and showed him the newspaper and brought to his attention the programmes that were on later. He seemed satisfied and we left asking him not to go out but to settle down to watch the TV. We explained that it would be Wednesday the next day as he kept asking. I wrote on the calendar when Matthew would be picking him up. (My eldest son and daughter-in-law had offered to take Dad for a few days over the holiday period for Alwyn and I to have a little break).

When we came home, I rang Ken to ask if he had brought his mother down to see Dad today, and he confirmed that it would have proved to be an impossible task due to her condition (Aunty Joyce is recovering from a stroke and is virtually immobile). Ken also stated that Dad had rung Aunty Joyce at 2am and 3.35am and accused her of 'playing tricks' on him with Gaynor. Of course, Aunty Joyce denied this and told Dad not to ring her again in the early hours of the morning. He was convinced that it was the afternoon and told her not to be so silly as 'Shirley would be up in a couple of hours to see me'. Ken and I both agreed that Dad's assessment needs to be brought forward and I said that I would speak to Bethan in the morning.

CHAPTER 5

Continued Confusion

29 December 1999 I spoke to Bethan and explained to her the events of the past two days. She said that, unfortunately, this kind of behaviour was quite common and because Dad was such an independent person there was no way that they would be able to take him into care at this stage. I said that the doctor had recommended that Dad was to have a brain scan to determine whether the drug 'Aricept' would be of benefit to him and also blood tests would be arranged by his own GP. Bethan advised that the appointment for 21st February 2000 was just a follow-up interview at Ysbyty Cwm Rhondda which did not involve the scan. The scan would have to be done in the new hospital and under the supervision of a different Consultant. Should the scan show that the drug would be likely to help Dad, then he would be strictly monitored, say every three months, to see how he was getting on. However, Bethan did stress that if this was the case, the drug merely 'puts a brake on' the situation for a while, but there is no cure for Alzheimer's Disease (at this point there was no definite diagnosis made). Bethan said that she would check with the doctor on his return to work on Wednesday, 5th January about the scan and would ring me to let me know what was happening.

4 January 2000 Dad rang at 00.35am asking if the nurse was coming today or tomorrow to take his blood pressure. I explained that he was ringing me in the early hours of the morning and not the afternoon! I told him to go back to bed and when he woke up in the morning it would be Tuesday and Bethan would be calling in the afternoon. Alwyn and I called in to see Dad at 6.30pm as usual and Bethan had left a note – there was no sign of Dad. He came back at 7pm and thought it was Wednesday morning.

5 January 2000 Bethan rang to say that she hadn't been able to get an answer at Dad's but she would arrange to call on him again to take his blood pressure. Bethan explained that it was her opinion (and stressed that it was only her thoughts on the matter) that Dad was likely to be having some very tiny strokes, not significant in size but very transient in nature and they would be enough to cause the confusion that Dad was experiencing. Unfortunately, if this is the case, then the drug Aricept would not be suitable treatment. However, it is just a matter of waiting until the scan has been done and the results made known before anything final can be said.

8 January 2000 Ken rang at 10.40pm – Dad had just arrived at Aunty Joyce's home, and as Ken was on very early morning shift, he wasn't able to bring him home. Alwyn and I went to fetch him and on our arrival, Dad was completely confused and bewildered. 'Is there anything wrong, Shirl?' he asked. When I said that I had come to take him back home, Dad became very annoyed and said that he'd only just got up to Aunty Joyce's. I gently explained that it was the night and not the morning and Ken also tried to reassure him, but Dad wasn't having any of it and blamed the Government for 'messing around with the clocks' and couldn't understand why we weren't confused as well! Dad then said that he wouldn't come up to see Aunty Joyce any more if it was causing problems. We lovingly explained to Dad that no-one was stopping him from coming up but it had to be in the day and not late in the night. He was, however, still not convinced and adamantly refused to visit again!

11 January 2000 We called at Dad's at our usual time and caught Dad coming out of his flat on his way out to do some shopping. He thought it was Wednesday morning. We took him back in and made him a cup of tea and showed him the News on the TV and reassured him with a gentle chat. We played cards, watched TV and left, reminding Dad not to go out again until it was light. I cried all the way home.

CHAPTER 6

The Clean-Up Campaign

21 January 2000 Gareth Morris (Social Services worker) made his first visit to Dad. Gareth's approach, like Bethan's, was very caring and professional. After the initial introductions, we sat down and discussed Dad's whole situation. At this point, it must be remembered that Dad was very much a fiercely independent person and was highly resistant to any thought of outside help. However, after a silent prayer (which in one form or another is being constantly made) Dad agreed to let me clean the living room next week! Thank You Lord for this little breakthrough.

28 January 2000 'First Big Clean' – Dad was hoovering when we arrived! Alwyn and I joined in and began the process of transforming the living room. We realized that it wasn't going to happen overnight, but the main thing was that we had made a start and Dad had agreed to our help! Praise the Lord.

31 January 2000 Dad's confusion over the telephone – he rang Myfanwy (Geraint's sister-in-law) who then rang me. I got through to Dad via the Operator. Dad must be pressing the wrong number. I rang Bethan to see if the scan could be brought forward as the initial request from the doctor had got lost in the post or during the transfer from the old hospital to the new hospital. Bethan said she would try, and gave our phone number to the hospital should a cancellation become available. Bethan also advised me that the specialist doctor was retiring and that Dad's case would be taken on by a new Consultant.

1 February 2000 Alwyn and I took Dad to see his GP as Dad really was in some discomfort with his leg again. The doctor examined him and said that some Tubigrip bandage would possibly help by supporting the leg in the daytime but that Dad was to take it off again in the night when he was in bed. Again, the doctor said that only an operation would be likely to benefit in the long run but that it was not advisable in Dad's case due to his age and also his longstanding condition of pneumoconiosis (coal dust on the lungs).

3 February 2000 I rang Dad at 6pm to ask how he was feeling and was met with another question – 'Who was that middle-aged man and ten year old child with you in my kitchen yesterday Shirley?' I said that I hadn't been to see him yesterday and confirmed that Alwyn and I would be up to visit him on Friday as usual. Dad was convinced that he had seen me and then reluctantly said, 'I must be seeing ghosts then!' I explained that he'd probably gone fast asleep and that he'd been having a very vivid dream. He said that it was the morning and that he'd just come in from doing the shopping.

4 February 2000 Gareth Morris called to see Dad today at 10.30am and there were some forms for Attendance Allowance to be completed. We discussed the possibility of our second 'clean-up campaign' and agreed to tackle the kitchen next. Gareth suggested that Dad help by cleaning the fridge by the next time he called and, because Dad tends to forget to do things, Gareth asked me to leave a note Sellotaped to the fridge as a reminder.

CHAPTER 7

Confusion, Delusion and Form Filling

8 February 2000 We visited Dad at our usual time – again he was quite convinced that it was the morning. He was totally confused and blamed the 'putting on and back the clocks for one hour' for his confused state. We tried to settle him by focusing his mind on playing cards but he was still unsure and wasn't entirely convinced of the right time. We left, assuring Dad that there was a good film on TV and asked him to stay in and watch it and not to go out any more this evening. We told Dad that the next day we would pick him up at 3.30pm to take him over to see the grandchildren and he seemed to be very pleased at the idea. Before we left, I arranged a whole set of clean clothes on the spare bed in readiness for Dad tomorrow.

9 February 2000 Dad was ready and eagerly awaiting our arrival – we were pleased to see that he had changed his clothes! As we were coming from the flat, I noticed Dad was limping and I asked him if he was alright. He said that he was but he had forgotten his walking stick. I went back in to fetch it and proceeded with our journey. Dad loved seeing the children and was quite pleased to see their progress. Toni (our second daughter-in law) made us a lovely meal and I could not help but notice how Dad was devouring his. When did he last eat properly?

13 February 2000 There was a phone call at 1.40pm whilst we were at Alwyn's mother's. It was Dad – he wanted to know why I had disappeared from his flat. He said that he'd been looking around the streets for our car but couldn't find it. I reminded him that it was Sunday and that we didn't usually visit him on this day and that we went straight from church up to Alwyn's mother's for lunch as we always did. He said that we called in to see him and then disappeared without a word. I reassured him that he must have been dreaming and asked him if he'd had his lunch. He said that he had and that he'd just made a cup of tea and that he was alright now that he knew where I was. There was no need for us to call in on him he said.

15 February 2000 A joint visit to Dad has been arranged today with Bethan and Gareth. Gareth commended Dad for cleaning the fridge. Dad said that he was upset about the fact that someone was telling him what to do by leaving such a note. Gareth apologized and said that it was just meant as a gentle reminder and not an official order! Later Gareth advised me that we would have to try and find another way of helping Dad to do things without making him feel upset and helping him to maintain a sense of dignity. Perhaps the approach could be to suggest he helps perform a task in order to help or alleviate some of the strain from me. In this way, he could perhaps be persuaded that he is taking more control of the situation rather than being told what to do. Bethan gently tried to persuade Dad to either have 'Meals on Wheels' or visit a Day Centre (she offered to arrange transport or take him herself) but he flatly refused to have anything to do with these options. Whilst on a previous visit, Bethan had noticed that Dad was experiencing some difficulty in lighting the fire and so she suggested that perhaps a change over to gas would help. I think I had better not put pen to paper as to what Dad's response was to that suggestion. Suffice it to say that he was not in favour! Bethan also tried to get Dad to consider a move to sheltered accommodation and suggested one of the local residences. There he would have people around for company (or privacy if he would prefer) but at least there would be a warden on hand in case of any emergencies etc. It would be nearer Porth – he could still do his own shopping and there would be no more trekking up through the Estate from the main road should he miss a bus. His response was, 'No way – it would be like living on a desert island! I don't want to be doing with all that moving nonsense – I'm too old for all that.'

Gareth had arranged for the DSS to send Dad an application form for Attendance Allowance and so I filled in the relevant part – Gareth completed his part and Bethan made a start on her part (medical). I suggested she completed it at our house as it was rather a lengthy form and Dad was getting a bit agitated by this time as he was having difficulty in hearing properly. We made arrangements for Bethan to take Dad to the Audiology Department at the Hospital on 3rd March. Bethan will be coming to our house with reference to the completion of the forms on 23rd February. (Forms need to be back in DSS by 6th March).

CHAPTER 8

Bad Leg and Baths

18 February 2000 Dad's birthday! Alwyn's mother and Dad came down for lunch and tea today. Although Dad knew it was his birthday (because of the cards through the post) he still seemed a bit bewildered on the day. We bought him an 'easy reader' watch that had large numbers, but he thought it was a mirror at first! Poor Dad. We gently showed him what it was and I undid the strap and put the watch on his wrist and indicated that it was more suitable than the one he was wearing as that had no numbers on it. He agreed and seemed to be very pleased with it. I just hope that it will be a means of help to him in assessing the right time of day. We all played cards which he likes to do even though he sometimes gets confused as to which game is being played and the order of play. During conversation, Dad complained of pain in his leg and he said he was sure it was to do with poor circulation of his blood. I asked him if he was having warm baths to relax his leg muscles and he said that he did so occasionally. Alwyn's mother asked Dad if he'd had the same problem whilst he was working, to which Dad replied, 'No – now you come to mention it – I don't think I did.' We suggested that perhaps the routine of an everyday shower (i.e. in the pit-head baths) could be substituted for an everyday bath at home to see if his situation would improve. Dad seemed very agreeable to this suggestion and appeared quite enthusiastic! So, if nothing else, hopefully at least Dad will be getting into some kind of routine with regard to his personal hygiene. I find it very difficult to broach this subject with him and so I have to jump at the opportunity when it arises and just encourage him to change his clothes every time he takes a bath. The day passed fairly well and after taking our visitors home, we came home and relaxed.

21 February 2000 Dad's concessionary coal arrived this morning. He rang at about 12.30pm to say that he had just finished putting the coal in. The coalman had only enough room to put two sacks in the coalhouse as it was full up. The remainder was dumped in the passage between the coal house and the kitchen and Dad was left to shovel the existing coal in the coalhouse further back in order to make room for the surplus (some further nine sacks!). My first reaction was to make a complaint to the relevant authority but when I mentioned it to Dad he told me not to make a fuss as he was alright. The driver had told Dad to burn more coal and then there would be sufficient room for him to put the whole delivery in the coalhouse and not leave it in the passage. I explained to Dad that I could ring the National Concessionary Coal Department and cancel the next load due in March (I did this with Dad's consent for December and January) and then, hopefully, this problem would not arise again. He agreed to this suggestion and I made a note to ring the Fuel Office.

22 February 2000 Dad appeared quite alert today and, although it seemed unfair for him to have put his load of coal in by himself yesterday, perhaps the extra bit of exercise had done him good. There was a marked improvement in his overall attitude and also his card-playing skills! For the first time in a long time, I came away from Dad's feeling a lot happier. Thank You Lord.

CHAPTER 9

Some Lost Things

23 February 2000 Bethan called this afternoon and together we completed the Attendance Allowance forms. I mentioned to Bethan that perhaps Dad was taking too much medication as regards his blood pressure tablets. If he had already taken his one tablet in the morning after breakfast as was his usual custom and practice, could it be possible that after taking a nap in the afternoon, on waking and thinking it was the morning, he could be taking another tablet following his second 'breakfast'? We already knew that on several occasions he has thought it was the morning and that he had just had his breakfast – so was it feasible to think that he'd taken his tablet as well? Of course, when we have explained that it is the evening, it is equally feasible to think that prior to going to bed/sleep in the night he would naturally take his night-time tablet. Bethan did say that there was a facility available from the chemist by way of a pack ready made up of daily doses of medication which could be delivered to the patient if required. On the other hand, it may be better if we could put his prescribed doses ready for him and then we would be in a better position to see if he was taking the correct amount per day. Bethan said she may have a suitable container at home which she could drop in to us tomorrow.

24 February 2000 Dad went to the Audiology Unit on his own – he had forgotten about the arrangements Bethan had made with him (which I'd written on his calendar). However, he did not have the complete hearing aid with him – only the part which houses the battery. He said he'd left the ear-piece on the table in the flat but when he came back home he couldn't find it. Unfortunately, the lady in the Audiology Unit couldn't help him other than give him a manual as to how to use the hearing aid. Regarding the 'lost' article, I suggested that I would help him to look for it when we came up next. I explained that perhaps when Bethan took him next week there might be something she could do if it hadn't been found by then.

25 February 2000 On visiting Dad this evening, he seemed quite depressed – he'd lost his bus pass. When I asked him when did he last remember using it, he said that he couldn't find it on the way home from the hospital yesterday. I said that perhaps someone had found it and handed it in to the Bus Depot if it had been dropped on the bus and, as it was too late to ring this evening, I would phone first thing in the morning. Dad told me not to bother as by now someone would have 'put their own photograph in and be using it for themselves'. However, I purposed in my heart to pray about the matter and see what would develop. We played cards but Dad didn't appear to be with us fully. We had a cup of tea with Dad before leaving. How I wish things were different!

26 February 2000 Dad rang this morning to say that his bus pass was found. Praise the Lord! He went on to explain that he got on the bus to Porth to do some shopping and told the bus driver that he had mislaid his pass. The driver suggested that Dad should go up to the Depot as it might have been handed in. Sure enough – there it was! Obviously Dad was very happy and he said, 'Well, Shirl, that's restored my faith in human nature' and said that the Lord had answered prayer. From the Depot, Dad went to the shops and had some lunch before going home. What a transformation from yesterday – I too was very happy for Dad. Thank You Lord for answering prayer yet again.

CHAPTER 10

Matters Medical and Legal

29 February 2000 The day of the CT Brain Scan. We called in at Dad's
at 1.30pm in plenty of time (appointment due 2.30pm) just in case
there was a problem i.e. Dad might have forgotten! However, we
were pleased to see that Dad had put on the clean clothes that I'd
laid out on the spare bed ready for him on Friday evening. He'd also
said that he'd taken a bath last night. There was some confusion,
however, as he had thought it was Sunday today. Then he seemed to
'come back to us' and was more orientated. In the car he showed
some apprehension as he had read in the local newspaper that
several old people had passed away recently and that they had been
patients in the same hospital to which we were taking him! I assured
him that he was simply going to the Radiology Department for a
special type of X-Ray which did not involve any kind of
injections/anaesthetic and that we would be back out within an
hour and that I would accompany him. Sure enough, as we were
early, Dad was called in at 2.10pm and was back out at 2.25pm! The
results will be sent to the new Consultant with whom we had an
appointment scheduled for 10.20am on Monday, 20th March.

On the way back home, we called in to the church where we were
celebrating our first anniversary of 'Young At Heart'. I introduced
Dad to quite a number of our group of elderly folk and he seemed to
be very shy in their company but, nevertheless, I hoped that
perhaps he may decide to come along with us on a weekly basis. We
can but hope!

2 March 2000 On Bethan's recommendation, Alwyn and I went

along to the local YMCA where a monthly meeting was being held by the Alzheimer's Society between 1pm and 3pm. There we met Lowri Jones who was able to give us very helpful advice and information in matters relating to caring for people with dementia. In particular, Lowri explained to us about the 'Enduring Power of Attorney' which would have to be applied for via a solicitor. This means that when Dad is no longer able to deal with financial matters himself then someone else can step in and take control. When we came home, I rang our solicitor to ask if she could point me in the right direction with regard to recommending a colleague who was sympathetic to the situation we were in, and who would be able to advise us accordingly. She highly recommended the services of her colleague in the same practice who had more experience in this particular field and she expressed her view that we were very sensible in our approach to the situation. After wishing us well she put us through to her associate. He was very polite and asked me a few preliminary questions. He asked me how many children Dad had and I explained that there was only my older brother who lived away and myself. He then arranged for us to have an appointment at 3pm on Wednesday, 8th March to discuss the situation.

I rang Derek to advise him on the developments and asked him if he would write a letter 'To Whom It May Concern' in order to pre-empt any questions that the solicitor may have with regard to responsibility for future events i.e. that Derek had no objections to me taking on the Enduring Power of Attorney. This seems to be a sensible solution in view of the fact that he is not on hand to deal with Dad's circumstances as they arise.

Dad rang Alwyn's mother at 10.30pm to ask if we were there as he was worried that we hadn't been up to visit him yet. He said, 'They usually come up at half past six and they haven't arrived yet and I'm getting worried, I hope and pray that they haven't been involved in a car crash – there's so much traffic on the roads these days!' Alwyn's mother explained that it was Thursday and not Friday and he seemed very surprised. She suggested that he should go to bed and not to worry as we would be up tomorrow as usual. After being reassured, Dad told Mam that he was experiencing some memory problems and that it was being looked into.

3 March 2000 I rang Dad to remind him that Bethan would be picking him up at 1.30pm to take him to the Audiology Unit to see about having a replacement hearing aid. He told me that 'it is written on the calendar!' and also mentioned the phone call to Mam last night. He asked me if we were going to the Memory Clinic next week and I advised him that our appointment was on 20th March. He is obviously concerned about his memory and so I think today may be the best time to broach the subject of the Enduring Power of Attorney. Bethan picked up Dad at 1.30pm and took him to the Audiology Unit as arranged. He had a fitting and was given a temporary hearing aid until his was ready. He paid for the replacement aid in cash (£51.00) and left the Unit and headed towards the bus stop in order to go home. Bethan had to go after him and remind him that she was taking him home.

As we called in this evening, Dad greeted us with the news that he'd been to 'order his new hearing aid' which had cost him £51.00. I immediately enquired as to how he had paid for it and he responded by saying, 'Well, er, um – I thought it would be about that much so I went to the bank yesterday to draw out some cash.' Somehow, his words didn't ring true and I had the feeling that he was carrying quite large amount of money in his wallet. If this was the case, then perhaps now was the time to discuss the issue of the EPA. I prayed that an opportunity would arise this evening – and sure enough it presented itself. Thank You Lord!

As the evening wore on, Dad told me that he'd received a letter from the Council advising him that he was in arrears with his rent. On checking the Council's statement with Dad's receipts, Alwyn and

I found the error. After a long discussion, I asked Dad if he would allow me to take over his financial affairs in order to alleviate himself and us from unnecessary worries. At first he was reluctant to 'put all this worry onto your shoulders' but I managed to convince him that because of his memory loss problems, it would be far better for me to handle his affairs once he became unable to make appropriate decisions for himself should the case arise. I gently explained that it was through no fault of his own that his memory was failing, but that it was due to his condition which would be discussed when next we saw the Consultant (20th March). Dad agreed that it would make sense to make the necessary arrangements now in the light of our discussion and so I told him that I would look into the legal situation next week and let him know my findings accordingly.

Dad still continues to be duped by the misguiding literature of the junk-mail conmen and persists in sending large amounts of money away. This has to stop or we will be back to square one again with arrears letters arriving on Dad's doormat. Before we left, I gave Dad some money towards paying off the rent arrears and he put the balance with it so that, once this amount was paid into the Post Office, the rent account would be cleared. I gave very specific instructions with regard to paying this money first thing in the morning and advised Dad to have a receipt and to ring me as soon as he came home. Dad apologized for 'all this trouble' and I said that, with the Lord's help, we would get things sorted out and for him not to worry. However, one incident that caused us concern was the fact that Dad opened the Parkray door and started to poke the fire which he had stacked too high with coal. This resulted in a live coal coming out onto the carpet as he was kneeling in front of the fire. Fortunately, we noticed it and so did Dad who managed to pick the coal up with the shovel and put it back on the fire. What Dad didn't notice, however, was that he had burnt a hole in his trousers and it was still burning! I quickly stopped the trousers from melting any further and, fortunately, no damage was done to Dad's leg. We asked Dad once again not to bank the fire so high and to keep it just level below the bars. He said he would watch that from now on! I just pray that he will take notice of our instructions as to how to keep the fire down to a more manageable level. Please Lord, keep Dad safe from danger.

CHAPTER 11

Night and Day Visits

4 March 2000 As there was no phone call from Dad today by 1.15pm, I rang to ask him if everything was alright at the Post Office. He seemed confused and unsure as to whether he'd had a receipt or not. I asked him to check and he said he would go down and have a chat with the man in the Post Office after lunch. As it happened, I rang the Post Office myself and spoke to a Mr Glyn James to explain the situation. He was very relieved that I had got in touch as both he and his wife were very concerned about Dad. Mr James knew that 'Mr Dowling had a daughter' as he had seen me on one occasion with Dad in the Post Office, but he didn't know how to get in touch with me to share his concerns regarding Dad. He explained that Dad's behaviour had changed considerably and that on several occasions Dad had called to the Post Office at 11pm and wanted to be served then. He thought that it was the morning and Mr James advised Dad to go back home to bed as it was getting very late. However, Dad insisted that he had to go to Porth to do some shopping. Eventually, Mr James was able to convince Dad that there would be no shops open at that time of night and persuaded him to go back home. Also, Mr James was concerned over the vast amount of money Dad was spending on sending money away to these rogues and said that although he could not stop him from purchasing the postal orders, he advised Dad not to send them by Registered Post, thus saving him £3.00 a time. Mr James said that he intended to speak to someone in Social Services to see if they could trace me to let me know what was going on. I explained the whole situation to Mr James including my intention to gain the Enduring

Power of Attorney on Dad's behalf and I thanked him very much for showing such great concern. He asked me for our telephone number so that he could contact us should the need ever arise. What a very understanding gentleman. Thank You Lord!

5 March 2000 I took Dad his lunch as arranged on the phone this morning, but he was sleeping in the chair when we arrived. As we avoid visiting Dad on Sundays due to our commitment to our church family and visiting my mother-in-law, perhaps we added to Dad's confusion. I feel guilty about 'having a break' from Dad but as Bethan said, I can't be with him 24 hours a day, seven days a week and I must have some time to myself – and look after myself as well! I have this sick feeling in my stomach all the time – I wish I could feel better. When Dad awoke, he thought we had come to fetch him to bring him down to our house and so I had to explain that it was not today that he was coming to visit. I felt so awful, especially when he went to the passage to put his hat and coat on. Dad said that his flat was always full of people coming to and fro – especially at this time of day. When I asked him, 'What people, Dad?' He replied, 'Oh I can't keep track of them all – lots of old women and children are constantly coming and going.' I explained that he had been sleeping when we arrived and that more than likely he had been having another vivid dream. However, he was adamant that these visitors were real people and wouldn't be persuaded any differently. I didn't pursue the matter because I had read in the literature that Bethan had given us that hallucinations were quite a common feature in people who suffered from dementia. I just made a note to remind me to let Bethan know what had happened. How I cried in the car on the way up to Alwyn's mother's home.

6 March 2000 I rang Dad to ask if he was alright and he said he was fine. I reminded him that it was my younger son's birthday tomorrow and, if he wanted to send Michael a card, then he could pick one up at the Post Office this morning after collecting his pension. He said of course he would like to send his grandson a card and asked me for his address. In case Dad might be found 'wandering' late in the night, I had taken the precaution of writing relevant names, addresses and phone numbers into a small pocket-sized book and advised him to keep it in his inside coat pocket. When I gently reminded him of the 'little book' he said, 'Of course! What is the matter with me!' Poor Dad, how I feel for him. The postmaster rang to say that Dad was trying to post a card but the address was incomplete on the envelope and asked me if I knew it. I explained that it was my son's birthday tomorrow and that Dad wanted to send the card. After giving the full address, I thanked Mr James for his kindness and concern and thought that was the end of the matter. I was wrong!

The phone rang at 11.50pm and I quickly got out of bed thinking there was an emergency. It was Dad! 'Shirl, I've been trying to get hold of our Michael but there's a woman on the end of the line saying "the number you have dialled has not been recognized – please check and try again" and she's getting on my nerves! I wanted to know if he'd received his birthday card. I know he's probably at work now, but I thought that Toni would be there to answer.' When I told Dad that Michael was probably in bed now as it was nearly midnight – he was amazed. I gave him the right number again and told him to ring tomorrow. 'You've been to work have you?' he asked and I said that I was going back to bed as I was having to get up at 4.30am. When it eventually 'got through' that it was very late in the night, Dad apologized for getting me out of bed and I said I would see him tomorrow at our usual time of 6.30pm.

7 March 2000 Dad seemed to be more 'with it' today and we actually played cards without too much repetition of the rules of play! On the subject of the Enduring Power of Attorney I told him that we had an appointment with the solicitor tomorrow at 3pm and we would pick him up at 2.15pm in plenty of time. I laid clean clothes on the spare bed in readiness for tomorrow's interview and also laid a clean bath towel on the bathroom chair suggesting he had a nice warm bath after we left. Dad thanked me for all my help and kissed me goodbye as usual.

8 March 2000 Dad rang about 11am and said that he'd had a visitor. Apparently someone was knocking at the door when he was in the bath. He got out of the bath, dressed and answered the door. On opening the door, he was greeted by a doctor who had come to examine him with regard to this 'emphysema business'. I asked Dad if he'd had an appointment in the post or by telephone saying when the examination was to take place. He said that the doctor told him that he was in the area and came 'on the chance' and that he was one of the doctors that had examined Dad on a previous occasion when he was called to a Medical Board in Cardiff many years ago. However the doctor said that he recognized Dad and told him to take his shirt off and proceeded to examine him. Dad had to blow into a type of tube (probably a spirometer) and then the doctor took a blood pressure reading and confirmed that it was OK. All fairly credible up to this point – although I was still a little sceptical. Then came the point where I began to believe that Dad was experiencing another hallucination. Dad said that the doctor had told him that he had put weight on since he examined him last! 'Do you really think so?' Dad asked. 'My daughter visits me regularly and she is concerned that I'm losing weight.' 'Oh no!' replied the doctor, 'you've definitely put weight on!'

At this point I told Dad to finish getting ready for our visit to the solicitor's office and that we'd be picking him up shortly. When I put the phone down, I explained to Alwyn what Dad had said and we both thought that it warranted investigation in case there was a bogus doctor in the area. You can never be too careful these days – particularly where there are elderly people who live alone. I checked with the solicitor who is handling Dad's compensation claim to see if there was a procedure in place for home visits by an appointed doctor in the case of claimants who were unable to attend the Medical Centre. The solicitor confirmed that there was such a procedure but that it was only carried out at the specific request of the claimant. She gave me a contact number to ring to find out if Dad had made such a request. On ringing, I was told that there was no such request on file and also no appointment arranged to visit Dad. In fact, Dad was not on their list at all for any such visit to perform a lung function test. I thanked them for their time and came to the conclusion that this was either a figment of Dad's imagination or a story he had made up to put my mind at rest regarding his weight situation!

We called for Dad this afternoon and took him to the solicitor's office as arranged. There we met Mr Jones who was most helpful in arranging for an office to be made available downstairs as he could see that Dad was using a walking stick and that his usual office (situated upstairs) might prove difficult to get to. I explained Dad's situation to Mr Jones and gave him Derek's letter 'To Whom It May Concern'. Dad was quite coherent and Mr Jones said that he had dealt with many cases like this and was very sympathetic without being patronizing. Mr Jones went on to say that Dad was being very sensible by allowing the Enduring Power of Attorney to pass to me under the circumstances. We then went on to provide Mr Jones with the necessary information that was required and left the office having made another appointment for next Tuesday in order to sign the official documentation. (Mr Jones had just made rough notes today prior to filling in the relevant forms). After sorting out the business, we thought it would be nice to take Dad over to see his great-grandchildren as he hadn't seen them for a little while. Of course he was pleased to see how much they had grown and he was quite happy playing with and chatting to them. Michael was sad to see how his Granddad was changing and he mentioned to me how he had noticed such a deterioration in his physical as well as mental condition. I explained that I was only recently coming to grips with the situation myself, and that as long as I kept reminding myself that it was Dad's illness that was making him like this, and I was not to take anything personally when he sometimes behaved in a way contrary to the way in which he would normally have done prior to becoming ill, then I was able to cope with it better.

Dad enjoyed a hearty meal and thanked Toni very much for such an excellent tea. Of course, we couldn't visit Michael and Toni without visiting Matthew and Pam (our elder son and his wife who live next door) and so it was more of the cups of tea and pancakes! Such hospitality – where were we going to find room in our stomachs? However, Dad not wanting to waste anything, managed along with us to make just enough room! As Matthew and Pam didn't know what to get Dad for his birthday, in the circumstances Pam suggested a bag of groceries. What a marvellous idea! In this way I could monitor Dad's eating habits without being too intrusive. After catching up on all the news, we took Dad home and put all the shopping away in the kitchen cupboard showing him where everything was. I showed him the frozen food which I'd put in the freezer and advised him to be careful to follow all the instructions as to how to prepare it. He said that it was very good of Matthew and Pam and appeared really grateful. Dad was very tired by this time and we advised him to go to bed and reminded him that we would be up on Friday at 6.30pm. Alwyn and I left feeling very worn out and ready for a bath and bed!

CHAPTER 12

More Junk Mail

10 March 2000 Dad rang at 8.35am saying that he'd received a letter advising him that he'd won £10,000 but in order to claim it he'd have to supply the company with his bank account details and National Insurance number. Both Alwyn and I explained in very strong terms that this was a con trick and that he should not divulge these details to anyone as there was a way in which these rogues could obtain credit cards and use them to run up huge debts which Dad would be liable to pay. We quoted an incident which appeared on TV quite recently in which a similar thing did happen and we strongly urged him not to give this important information away. Dad said that he understood and promised not to reveal these details and was grateful to us for pointing the matter out to him. We called in to see Dad this morning before going up Alwyn's mother's and Dad was sorting out some junk mail envelopes. He said that he was fed up with receiving such mail and also said that he was going to write a letter to them saying he no longer wished to receive their mailings. I suggested that I type some letters out for him to sign on Tuesday when we came up and he agreed that it would be a good idea. He said it would look more professional and perhaps they would take more notice of a typed rather than a hand-written letter. As he was going to Porth for his lunch, we gave him a lift to the main road where he wanted to go to the Post Office first. We continued on our way letting Dad know that we would be up to see him later at 6.30pm. Dad appeared quite well this evening and we played cards as usual. He seemed very focused and we noticed that he was playing very craftily and as a result won every game! He was certainly 'with it' tonight. We had a cup of tea with him, watched some TV and reminded him that we were due to go to the solicitor's office on Tuesday morning. I wrote the details on his calendar and said that I'd be in touch before then to remind him. He seemed to be alright with that, and so Alwyn and I made our weary way home!

11 March 2000 Dad rang to say that he'd received an acknowledgement letter from the DSS in relation to his claim for Attendance Allowance. Alwyn took the call as I was resting and Dad said that the letter stated 'we may need more information from you'. After listening to the whole letter being read out, Alwyn assured Dad that it was a standard letter that was issued to everyone who had put a claim form in for this allowance and there was no need for a reply. Dad accepted the explanation and told Alwyn to 'let Shirley know when she wakes up but don't disturb her now'. Dad seems to be more himself today.

13 March 2000 1.30pm. I rang Dad to remind him we were going to see the solicitor tomorrow and asked him to put some clean clothes ready. He said that he'd fetched his pension and gone to Porth and had lunch in the Café. 'Very good' I thought, 'at least he's having something substantial to eat instead of snacking on biscuits!' I told him that I was pleased that he'd had a nice lunch and I also reminded him that I'd typed up the letters he wanted. 'What letters, love?' he asked. 'The ones to stop the junk mailings,' I said. He'd forgotten!

9.30pm. Dad rang and was very upset – 'Shirl, is that you? Thank God – I've been going out of my mind with worry – I've imagined all sorts of things!' I told him to keep calm and asked him what the trouble was. 'You are late picking me up I thought your car had taken a bump and you were involved in a road accident.' When I explained that it was still Monday, he couldn't believe it. He said his clock was showing half past ten and I asked him to press the 'speaking clock' button whilst I was on the phone to him (the clock is on the table near the phone so I knew that I'd be able to hear the 'voice' loud and clear). 'Nine thirty-six pm!' rang out and so I explained to Dad that it was night time and that I was getting ready for bed. I suggested that he did the same and assured him that both Alwyn and I were fine and that we would be up to see him in the morning. Dad was very relieved and apologized for disturbing us. I told him not to worry and that we would be picking him up tomorrow as planned.

14 March 2000 9.00am. Dad rang with regard to junk mail 'winnings' (convinced he'd won again!).

9.30am. We arrived at Dad's and after reading the letters explained yet again that it was a con. This was borne out by a newspaper article which we brought to Dad's attention. However, he said that this was the last time he was sending off money and if he didn't hear anything then he would write a letter to our local newspaper warning other people about it! (He would then sign and send off my typed letters – or so he said – we'll see!).

10.50am. We arrived at the solicitor's and Dad and I signed the official paperwork in relation to the Enduring Power of Attorney. No problems there. However, on the way out of the office, I asked Mr Jones if it was now possible for me to arrange for Dad's mail to be re-directed to our address as there was quite a volume of junk mail coming through his letter-box which I wanted to stop. He said that I could set the wheels in motion for whatever was needed with regard to Dad's best interests. Should there be a problem in the meantime, I was to advise people that the application for the EPA was going through and I was to give his telephone number in case of any queries. Notices of application would be sent out shortly and it would take between six and eight weeks for things to be finalized with the registration process at the Public Trust Office. I thanked Mr

Jones for dealing with this matter so sympathetically and for making things so easy for us.

We brought Dad back to our house where I gave him his first lesson in microwave cooking! Chicken dinner with all the trimmings no less! Dad was over-awed at how quickly his lunch cooked and he said that it 'was very tasty indeed!' We said that should he be successful with his claim for Attendance Allowance then we would get him a microwave oven and he appeared quite enthusiastic. A breakthrough. (If not successful, I'll see what we can arrange between us). Dad mentioned in passing that he'd cleaned the top of his cooker yesterday as it may be a fire-risk if the excess hardened cooking fat caught alight when the ring was turned on. I praised him for his efforts and told him that I was pleased that he'd remembered to do this task without me having to prompt him! Thank You Lord – Your hand is near. After lunch, we played cards and all went fairly well. We took Dad home before going up to see Alwyn's mother and reminded Dad strongly that we wouldn't be up this evening at our usual time of half past six in case he was worried as to our whereabouts again. I said that we would be up on Friday. He seemed to understand. Please look after him in the meantime Lord – I know that You are in control of every situation. Thank You.

CHAPTER 13

The 'Burglar Shift'

15 March 2000 6.00pm I rang Dad – no answer.

6.10pm I rang Dad – no answer.

6.20pm I rang Dad – no answer.

6.30pm I rang Dad – Dad answered! What a relief – thank You Lord. I thought Dad had gone out shopping again but he said he didn't hear the phone ringing as he'd only just got up from bed. He said that he'd gone into the living room and someone had already lit the fire but assured me – 'It wasn't me!' I said that he'd lit the fire earlier on in the day and now it was evening. Again, he was really confused and thought that it was morning and that he was just about to go to the shop for his newspapers. Thankfully I managed to convince him that it really was the evening and told him to look at his newspaper that he'd already bought to see what programmes were on tonight. As he likes 'Coronation Street' I reminded him that it would be on later tonight because there was a football match on. Once again I reminded him not to take his medication yet as it was too early, but instead to take his tablets before going to bed later on. This constant reminding must be so wearing for Dad as he is so bewildered by what is happening to him! Poor Dad, I just pray that he will be able to settle into some sort of routine soon. I said that I would phone him again tomorrow to see how he was.

16 March 2000 Alwyn and I came home from having our hair cut this afternoon and I pressed the 1471 number on the phone to see if anyone had rung whilst we were out. As it happened, Dad had rung at 16.06. I called back and asked Dad if he was alright. 'Nothing's wrong Shirl, I'm just ringing to ask if it's today that we're going to the Memory Clinic. Only I'm going on what you wrote on my calendar.' I explained that we still had a few days to go yet as we were due to go on Monday. 'Well it's Monday today isn't it? I was just about to go down to the Post Office to fetch my pension!' Again I explained the days of the week to him and told him that it was Thursday today. 'Well, they're mixing up the days on the calendar as well now are they? I don't know – I don't know what the world is coming to – it wasn't like this when I was a boy. Why don't they leave things alone?' There was just no reasoning with Dad and I decided to try and change the subject (by this time we had been on the phone for almost an hour!). 'Well, Dad, if you go out again this evening, you will be doing "the burglar shift",' I said. This was a phrase Dad used when he was working in the colliery when he referred to the night shift which he used to hate to work! I thought he might identify with this phrase and cause him not to go out when it was dark – who knows – it might work! Once more I assured him that I was ringing him to try and get him back into line as far as the right time of day or night was concerned and that it was not for the purpose of checking up on him or invading his privacy. Dad said that he was grateful for what I was doing and I expressed the hope that when we saw the Consultant and had the result of the scan that a way may be found to alleviate some of his confusion. We continue to pray. I reminded Dad that it was Friday tomorrow and that we would be up to visit him as usual after we had visited Alwyn's mother.

17 March 2000 The mystery of the 'doctor's visit' on 8 March was uncovered this evening. Dad was right after all and we were wrong! A doctor did actually call on Dad to give him a medical examination at home – it was in connection with his existing entitlement to Industrial Injuries Benefit. He showed us a letter which he received from the DSS giving him the results of his 'Board'. Well, you could have knocked us down with a feather! Dad's story was so believable up to the point of the comment, 'You've put weight on since I saw you last' that we assumed wrongly that Dad's visit by a doctor was all in his mind. This comment, along with the absence of an appointment letter and there being no record of Dad's details for a house call by the solicitor's Medical Appointee, led us to believe that this event was hallucinatory in nature rather than an actual event. However, there were still some things that needed to be confirmed and I made a note to speak to Dad's solicitor on Monday.

CHAPTER 14

The Scan Results

20 March 2000 Alwyn and I arrived at Dad's at 9.20am. He was ready and eagerly awaiting his appointment. As we had a few minutes to spare before leaving, I rang the DSS regarding Dad's 'Board'. As it happened, there was no cause for alarm as the claim in question was for Dad's existing, long-standing claim for pneumoconiosis. It had nothing to do with the matter regarding emphysema and the letter was just to advise Dad that he was eligible to receive his 'dust money' for life as no further examinations were necessary. The award figure payable weekly represented the 10 per cent loss of lung function due to the pneumoconiosis. Phew! With that matter sorted out, there was no need for me to ring the solicitor. Now on to the most important appointment of the day after explaining the situation to Dad.

We arrived at the hospital at 10.10am. I asked Bethan if she would sit in on the consultation as she is already based at Ysbyty Cwm Rhondda and her care for Dad throughout since the day she became involved has been wonderful. Obviously, I asked Dad if he minded this and he said that he had no objections – in fact he was quite happy about it.

The new Consultant introduced himself to us and there was plenty of room for everyone to sit down. It was just as well – the CT scan results had finally come through and, although I had steeled myself for this moment, I couldn't help but feel that the news we were about to hear was best heard if we were sitting down. However, it came as no great shock in one way because we already had some inclination as to what was happening to Dad by way of Bethan's possible explanations all along. Nevertheless, the words were now becoming fact and it took a great deal of concentration to take in what the doctor was saying. The scan showed that there were two areas in Dad's brain that were showing signs of damaged cells – the areas concerned with memory and speech. This was due to lack of oxygen going to the brain via the arteries and so, effectively, these brain cells were being cut off from the supply and as a result, these cells eventually die. There is no cure for this ageing process, but the doctor said that new drugs were being tested and possibly by the time he sees Dad next (in six months) there may be a drug on the market that may be of some help. However, on reviewing Dad's medication prescribed by the GP, the Consultant felt that the dosage of aspirin Dad was taking appeared to be on the high side and so he was going to ask the reason for it with the view to amending it. His advice was to stay with the prescribed dose unless otherwise notified. I explained that we were concerned with the irregularity in the way Dad takes his tablets and how he becomes confused over day and night, and may therefore be taking too many inadvertently. Again, as Bethan explained, 'George still refuses any outside help such as a Carer to come in once a day and Shirley lives at quite a distance, so is unable to visit on a daily basis to administer or supervise his medication.' Dad, it must be said, is his own worst enemy! Things could be so much easier in one respect if only he would 'bend' just a little. He still has that stubborn streak. I don't blame him one bit for wanting to keep his independence, but I just wish that he would help himself by allowing someone to help him! Please, Lord, will You open up the way? On the positive side, Dad heard this week that he'd been granted the Attendance Allowance. This means that we can make Dad's life a bit more comfortable and go ahead with the purchase of a microwave cooker. Another point to note is that because Dad is now officially recognized as a person with mental impairment, then he no longer has to pay the Council Tax. The doctor signed the certificate which I have to present to the local Council Authority. From this day on, Dad is exempt from this payment. It has to be said that Dad emphasized time and time again that the Attendance Allowance should have been in my name because I was looking after him and doing his washing and taking him to hospital and solicitor's appointments etc. I explained to Dad that all we needed was 'a fiver now and again for the petrol and a packet of washing powder'.

Alwyn and I sorted out some of Dad's business after taking him home and we eventually got home about four o'clock feeling rather the worse for wear! However, it must be noted that throughout this whole experience, the prayers of our church family were being felt as we were comforted by the thought that people cared enough to set time aside to pray for us when, perhaps, sometimes we couldn't pray for ourselves. As someone once said – 'God is good – all of the time!'

CHAPTER 15

Angels and Clocks

21 March 2000 We had just settled down to a cup of tea with Dad when there was a knock at the door. When I answered it a young man asked if he could have a word with me. I said, 'Of course' and he beckoned me to come up to the garden gate where his wife and child were. He said that he thought I should know that they found Dad standing by the gate at about half past nine on Sunday night, anxiously waiting for me. It so happened that the lad, Huw, knew Matthew and Michael from former schooldays. Huw said that he and his wife, Cerys, knew we visited Dad every week but asked, did we know that he was out wandering the streets in the early hours of the morning? I explained Dad's condition and they said they were very sorry and that they would 'keep an eye open' for him. Huw and Cerys live in the upstairs flat opposite Dad and so I thanked them very much for their concern. The Lord has His angels everywhere! I went back into Dad's flat and just said that the young lad across the road saw Alwyn and me coming up and wanted to say 'Hello' and to make himself known as Matthew and Michael's friend at football/ school. 'Small world, isn't it?' said Dad.

We didn't have a very long time to play cards tonight, but it was just as well as I wanted to change the bedclothes and wash the bath before going home. Dad's fire seems to be 'choked up' again tonight! No hot water – as there's no air getting to the back of the fire to heat up the boiler. Back to 'Smokey Joe's'! Once again I reminded Dad gently that he must not have the coal banked up quite so high. There's a real possibility of a live coal coming out onto the carpet if he's not careful. He said he'd try and remember next time. How sorry I feel for this man who was once my father. Here's me telling him how to light and keep a fire going when, once upon a time, I was taking advice from him as to how to perform this very same task! It's so very sad . . . Alwyn and I left and Dad carried the bags of washing to the car – he wants to feel that he still can be of some use, bless him. Oh Lord – what's going to become of him?

23 March 2000 I rang Dad to remind him that it was Kiara's birthday on Sunday (his great grand-daughter's first birthday) and if he would like to send a card, then the address was in the little book of names and addresses that I'd written out for him previously. I advised him not to go out again today as it was getting late and also it was raining quite heavily. 'If you write the details down on a separate piece of paper, Dad, you can then take it with you to the Post Office tomorrow and buy a suitable card and post it off for it to arrive on Saturday.' He seemed happy with that suggestion but then he said, 'See you later on then love,' and thought that it was Friday afternoon! Once again I explained that it was Thursday today and that we wouldn't be up until tomorrow. He seemed so bewildered and said rather pathetically, 'I don't know what's the matter with me these days, Shirl. It seems as if I'm out of tune with the rest of the world.' I tried to reassure him and told him that we were going to try to make his physical life a little more easier and more comfortable. We bought Dad his microwave cooker today and said we'd be up tomorrow to show him how it works.

24 March 2000 As it happened, Alwyn and I called to Dad's first thing this morning to deliver the microwave cooker and return his clean washing to save us carrying them around in the car with us all day. Dad hadn't gone out by 9.30am (which is highly unusual!) and so we left everything in the spare bedroom until we came back this evening. Friday is our busiest day but we gave Dad a lift to Porth before visiting our two elderly ladies in the church and also Alwyn's mother. We reminded Dad as we dropped him off that we would be calling back at our usual time of half past six. He seemed happy – and off he went! However, when we arrived at Dad's at 6.20pm – there was no sign of him!

This time the kettle was not warm (neither was the teapot nor the toaster). His overcoat and walking stick were missing from the passage which probably meant that he had gone 'on his travels' again or that he hadn't yet come back from this morning. I decided not to panic but to pray! In the meantime, I took advantage of the fact that Dad wasn't in and managed to do some cleaning in the kitchen and the bathroom. However, the time was now getting on and by about eight o'clock I started to get a bit anxious as there was still no sign of Dad. Alwyn had fixed a digital clock on the wall above the telephone so that Dad could look at it whenever he was unsure of the day etc as this particular clock displays details of the day of the week, the actual time (12 hour display as opposed to the 24 hour display) and also the date. So, when Dad came home at 8.10pm we asked him if he was alright and where had he been until such a late hour. He said that he'd gone to Porth and that there were no buses coming back up so he started to walk. Someone took pity on him and brought him home to the gate. I explained to Dad how worried we were getting and he said that he didn't realize it was getting so late and thought he would be back before we arrived for our visit. Then we showed him the digital clock on the wall and asked him to tell us what time it was displaying. After a while, he could recognize the day and time etc and marvelled at the technology that enabled all the information to be displayed in such a way. Reminding him over a nice hot cup of tea, we said for him to check on the clock if ever he was pondering over what day it was, so that hopefully, his confusion might be lessened a little bit. We can but try! Before leaving, we showed Dad how to use the microwave cooker – his second lesson – and kept things very basic. He enjoyed his Irish stew supper and again marvelled at the technology involved. He hugged me and I said I'd ring him tomorrow. We came home exhausted!

25 March 2000 I rang Dad as promised and, at 11.30am was surprised to have an answer! He was listening to the radio programme 'String of Pearls' which plays all the old familiar tunes which 'bring back lots of memories'. He said that the tunes were making him cry and I said that, although it was nice to hear the music, if it was causing him to be depressed, then he shouldn't really dwell on things in such a melancholy way as it may prove to be too upsetting for him. He agreed to some extent but I had the feeling that he was beginning to have his own little 'pity party' and 'I'm feeling sorry for myself' time and so I tried to encourage him not to focus too much on the negative side of things but to concentrate on the things that he could still do, i.e. go out shopping, do some household chores etc. I reminded him that the clocks should be put forward one hour this weekend and that we'd come up Sunday night after visiting Alwyn's mother in order to make sure that all his clocks and watches were showing the correct time. As in the case of any suggestion to change his coal central heating to gas, I had better not put pen to paper with regard to Dad's response to the changing of the clocks!

CHAPTER 16

Almanacs and Anthracite

26 March 2000 Dad was totally confused this evening! Even more so than usual. He asked how many 27ths there were in one month and when I replied, 'Only one', he said that his calendar was all wrong! He'd gone to the Post Office this morning, thinking it was Monday and was quite aggrieved that the Postmaster wouldn't give him his pension. I gently explained that it was Sunday and that the Post Office did not open on Sundays, but he said that he saw Mr James coming back after doing a night shift of selling ice-cream. Be that as it may (or may not be!) I explained that his pension was not due until tomorrow, to which he replied that 'the whole world is going haywire – I don't understand it!' Poor Dad, he feels that the whole world is confused and that he is the only one who has the right angle on things. It must be so frustrating for him. 'This is like Chinese to me,' said Dad, referring to the large squares on his calendar. He doesn't appear to be able to follow the days or the months now – even though there is only one page to one month. How sad is the effect of this dreaded dementia – the illness that no-one can put a plaster on with the hope of getting better.

After a while Dad said that Aunty Joyce had been down to see him and that he'd made her a cup of tea. It was still on the table with a saucer over it to keep it warm. He said he thought Aunty Joyce had gone to the bathroom and then gone home without saying a word. The coal fire was still causing a problem. Dad will not entertain the thought of changing over to any other method of heating, and so we battle on wrestling with the poker and trying to draw the fire up in order for there to be hot water for a bath etc.

I explained to Dad that he must not put empty plastic milk containers onto the fire to help it to light as this gives off poisonous fumes and causes the room to be filled with toxic black smoke. I stressed that it was vitally important to stop doing this as he had enough problems with pneumoconiosis without making the situation worse. He said that he didn't realize that it would cause such a problem as I was explaining, and he assured me that he wouldn't do it again. Eventually, we managed to get the fire to draw properly and the radiator in the kitchen became hot. 'The first time in a long time,' Dad said.

During our visit Dad said that he was having pain in his knee and that it was very uncomfortable at times. I suggested that I make an appointment with Dad's GP with a view to having a check-up. He flatly refused and went on at some length about the problems caused by aspirin which he'd read about in the paper. Alwyn explained that the aspirin that Dad was taking was the 'coated' type which were quite safe – but Dad wasn't having any of it and said so in not so many words! 'He'll only give me something else which won't cure my knee or varicose veins, so I don't want to bother at all with the Doctor – so leave it there!' What am I to do if Dad won't co-operate? It's so very difficult! I gave him two paracetamol tablets for the pain and filled a hot water bottle to place it on his knee to see if that would give him some relief as well. When the water was warm enough, I suggested that perhaps a nice soak in the bath might be of some help. It wouldn't hurt him anyway. We altered the clocks and Dad's watch before leaving and gave him another lesson on microwave cooking (again, keeping things very basic) and he said that he'd 'have a go tomorrow'. I said I'd phone him to ask him how he got on and reminded him that we'd be up on Tuesday evening as usual. I still continue to trust God, even though sometimes I cannot understand the way He is taking us through this trial. My faith is strong, despite the circumstances, and I'm convinced that the trials of life are intended to make us better not bitter! Thank You Lord.

CHAPTER 17

Avoiding Confrontation

27 March 2000 I rang Dad this morning and he seemed quite 'chirpy'. He'd been to collect his pension and he sounded on top form! When I asked him what he'd bought by way of shopping, he replied, 'Food, of course!' That told me didn't it? When I further asked if he'd used the microwave cooker today, the reply came back quick as a flash, 'Yes – I had a couple of pennyworth of it today – very nice too!' I then asked him how his knee was and he said he was getting more relief from applying the hot water bottle than 'any of those tablets – they're not a bit of good!' Afraid to ask Dad any more questions, I told him that I was glad he was feeling a bit better today and that Alwyn and I would be up to see him tomorrow at our usual time of 6.30pm.

28 March 2000 Not a lot to report today – pretty average sort of interaction as we've experienced in time past, i.e. confusion over time of day etc. I'm beginning to learn how to deal with this situation by avoiding any kind of confrontation with Dad as he feels the whole world has 'gone haywire' (his own words not mine). I gently move on by changing the subject and diverting his attention to something else. He's quite forgotten the earlier conversation by the time we discuss another topic. After playing cards, I showed Dad how to cook a jacket potato in the microwave and he appeared to grasp the idea. I said that I'd get him some cooked dinners by the end of the week so that he'd have a variety of foods that just needed to be cooked for about ten minutes. This way, I will be able to monitor his eating habits and see if he is eating properly when we're not there. Dad said he would like to have these meals rather than 'Meals on Wheels'.

29 March 2000 9.45am. I rang Dad to see how things were today. He had been down to the Post Office and paid his phone bill as I had explained to him last night. However, he went to Porth to pay his bill and when I said that he could pay it at the same time he picked up his Industrial Injuries Benefit, Dad told me that he didn't want to do that. He said that the postmaster was 'funny with me yesterday and wouldn't give me my money.' Dad went on to say that Mr James didn't give him his money because it wasn't due yet for payment. Of course, Mr James was quite right to decline Dad's request as it was the wrong day, but when I explained this to Dad he said, 'Well, it was only the case of a few hours and it would save me having to go to the Post Office again tomorrow'. 'It doesn't work like that, Dad', I explained, 'what if everybody tried to claim their Benefits a day too soon? There would be no money left in the Post Office to carry on with everyday transactions!' 'I suppose you're right, love, but anyway – I went to Porth instead to pay the phone bill after that.' Oh well! We can but plod on! I said I'd ring him this evening.

30 March 2000 When I phoned this morning, I reminded Dad to leave the fire go out at the end of the day so that we could go up tomorrow morning to service the Parkray. Alwyn and I were taking a break and going to Llantwit Major for the day. When we came home, I rang Dad once again to see how he was and also to give him another prompt to let the fire go out tonight. 'What do you mean?' he said, 'Aren't you coming up now to do the fire – it's all ready for Alwyn to sort it out now. You told me yesterday to let the fire go out and I've done it and cleared out all the ashes for him.' I explained that I rang this morning at 9.45am not yesterday. Dad became quite cross and said, 'I won't argue with you, Shirl, but you did phone me yesterday – if I don't move from this chair!' Well, not wanting to get into a confrontational situation, I apologized that we weren't able to come up at that moment but I advised him to keep warm by having a hot cup of tea and by going to bed as it was getting late. I said that we would be up as soon as possible on Friday morning and reminded him to look at the clock under the picture on the wall by the phone whenever he wanted confirmation of the time of day and also the day of the week. Dad seemed to calm down after reassurance that we'd be up the next day.

31 March 2000 4.30am. Alwyn and I got up for work as usual – only this time it was different. This was to be our last day of working part-time and it's not before time. We are both feeling the strain of trying to come to terms with juggling with our own health problems, those of Dad and working part-time for five days a week. So it is with a feeling of relief that we look forward to today!

Work over, back home, change our clothes, up to Dad's, change, clean the kitchen and bathroom, service the Parkray, wash, change, give Dad instructions on microwave cooking for his lunch, supervise him whilst he is operating the microwave cooker, pick up Dad's laundry, visit Alwyn's mother, have lunch, drop Alwyn's mother at the bingo hall, back home, put Dad's washing in, have a bath, supper, bed. Goodnight!!!!

CHAPTER 18

Brief Observations

Of course, it would be impossible for me to relate every minute detail as to the effect that this illness is having on both Dad and ourselves as a family, but it may be helpful for the reader to note some of the symptoms that presented themselves during the next six months.

2 April 2000 Difficulty in dealing with the front door lock from the inside (previously would have been able to understand the workings of the lock).

7 April 2000 Accidental fall at home resulting in injury to forehead – hospital treatment required.

12 April 2000 Concerns regarding weight loss. Average weight previous year, approximately 10st 7lb - 11st, current weight 9st 5lb.

21-23 April 2000 Continued confusion over days, times etc. Medication for whole week taken in three days.

28 April-12 May 2000 Admission to hospital for two weeks' respite care.

19-22 May 2000 Medication for whole week taken in four days.

23 May 2000 Social Services assessment carried out regarding the necessity of Home Care supervision of medication morning and evening.

24 May 2000 Accidental fall outside home (near main road) resulting in minor abrasions to forehead.

29 May 2000 Delusions regarding his flat not being his own home – 'Can you fetch me and take me to the other Shrewsbury Avenue?'

2 June 2000 Visited his sister-in-law in Ystrad at 9am leaving his front door ajar and his side door closed but unlocked. Also, left home prior to Carer's arrival.

6 June 2000 Late night wandering in Porth.

7 June 2000 Another early morning visit to his sister-in-law. He was inappropriately dressed (underwear worn on top of his trousers).

16 June 2000 Inappropriately dressed – trousers on inside out.

26 June 2000 Lost front door key.

7 July 2000 Cancelled assessment with Social Services with reference to Home Care help to manage the fire. Insisted he could manage on his own and that it was 'not women's work!'

13 July 2000 Assessment with Ysbyty Cwm Rhondda Day Care Unit staff at home. He presented very well (probably due to the fact that he had been reminded several times of the forthcoming visit!).

21 July 2000 Late night local wandering – brought home by family member.

25 July 2000 Social Services assessment with reference to suitability for attendance at Day Centre for the 'elderly and frail'. Arrangements made for volunteer transport to and from venue.

29 July 2000 Inability to recognize his son at first who had come to stay with him for a week. Dad was alright after it was explained to him that it was a surprise visit. (They last saw each other two years ago).

1 August 2000 Tried to fill the toaster with water thinking it was the kettle.

2 August 2000 Insisted on going out 'to do some shopping in Porth' despite his son's pleading with him to stay at home because it was very late in the night. Came back after an hour or so.

4 August 2000 First visit to Day Centre – mediocre response.

8 August 2000 Late afternoon 'visit to sister-in-law' but, on checking it was found that he hadn't been there at all. Came home soaking wet due to the weather.

11 August 2000 Second visit to Day Centre – very adamant he does not want to go there again ('too noisy').

18 August 2000 Crisis phone call 6.30am. Parkray glass broken – live coals on carpet. Emergency call-out for Council contractor to repair damaged glass front. Social Services assessment arranged for safer form of heating to be installed.

1 September 2000 Picked up at 8.30pm by Home Care worker. Although she managed to persuade him to go home to take his evening medication, he was insistent that he wanted to go out again to find his home. He became quite aggressive and accused the Home Care worker of burning his slippers on the fire as he couldn't find them.

5 September 2000 'On the hop' visit by Ysbyty Cwm Rhondda Day Care Unit staff. Dad very disoriented.

13 September 2000 First visit to the Ysbyty Cwm Rhondda Day Care Unit – more comfortable response – seemed much happier with the environment there than in the previous Day Centre.

16 September 2000 Dad was very depressed today – he confessed to crying his heart out. He insists that other people have been in his flat and disturbing things such as his newspapers. He says that he'll have to find 'another hiding place for them'.

17 September 2000 Dad confessed to feeling much better this morning. However, by late afternoon, early evening he was convinced that Alwyn had been in his flat and that he'd been talking with him. He was also convinced that Alwyn had seen to his fire and that it was now drawing up well! When it was explained that Alwyn hadn't been there at all that day, Dad became quite aggressive over the phone and very annoyed to think that he was 'being told fibs'. There was just no reasoning with him – he was adamant and did not want to believe that there was a medical problem which was causing these delusions. He flatly refused to be reassured.

General Comments

Generally speaking, over the past six months my family and I have seen quite a rapid change for the worse in my father's condition. We have come to notice that at times his behaviour is quite out of character. He becomes very moody and aggressive if things are not 'going his way' and tends to take it out on whoever is the nearest to him at the time. For instance, it has been reported to me by neighbours that when someone has kindly let him know which bus stop to get out at, he in no uncertain terms has told them to mind their own business and has become verbally abusive. He is usually very polite and does not resort to bad language. He has also become increasingly forgetful (more so than previously) to the point of buying the same newspapers three or four times in the same day. He continues to be delusional as regards people 'visiting' such as his sister-in-law for whom he constantly makes tea and sandwiches. He is also unable to recognize close family members' photographs.

CHAPTER 19

The Next Step

It is with a heavy heart that I write concerning the outcome of Dad's second assessment with the Consultant Psychiatrist at Ysbyty Cwm Rhondda on Monday, 18 September 2000. It was evident from the discussions that Dad had now moved into another stage of the dementia i.e. from the mild stage to the moderate stage. Although I recognize and acknowledge the fact that Dad's condition is getting worse, it's the speed at which it is developing that is taking me by surprise. Nevertheless, I am fully persuaded that whatever happens, the God that I serve will take care of my father. It just sometimes takes a little time to adjust to what is actually happening. However, without my faith in God and the strong support of my husband and sons, along with members of my church family, the strain of looking after Dad would have been too much for me to bear.

So it is then that I continue to write these extracts from my diary with the view to giving the reader a little more insight into the daily goings-on in the life of both the 'Cared For' and the 'Carer' so that, hopefully, they may be of some help to others who may be found in a similar situation.

20 September 2000 Dad rang early to say that he had bad news – his Grandmother had died during the night and his mother had come to the bedroom to let him know. (His mother was supposed to be one of the people in charge of 'this place'). I assured him that he had been dreaming as his Grandmother had died many years ago when I was a child. I said that we would be up shortly to take him to the new Day Centre. He was still unconvinced that he'd been dreaming and when we got to the Day Centre, I explained the situation to one of the members of staff in case he became agitated because he felt he needed to go to the funeral. He was settled in with a cup of tea and introduced to some activities which, for a while, seemed to take his mind off things. However, when Alwyn and I came to fetch him home, Dad still wondered if we ought to let Gaynor know about the funeral arrangements. Once again I reassured him that everything was alright and he appeared to be OK as we left, promising to return on Friday as usual.

22 September 2000 Today is Friday and, thankfully, no more has been mentioned by Dad regarding his Grandmother. I feel it is best if we do not say anything about Wednesday's episode as, quite frankly, it seems as if it's a forgotten incident. It is so very wearing emotionally to go through the same explanations time and time again whilst still keeping a calm posture. So, 'Thank You Lord for Your help once again.'

26 September 2000 The Community Occupational Therapist is due to call to Dad today at 2pm in order to assess the need for a safer form of central heating. The interview went well and Nia Edwards expressed her support in such an empathetic way as she was speaking from personal experience. Unfortunately, her mother suffers with the same complaint as Dad and so she had great insight into our situation. Dad, by this time, is now acknowledging the fact that he cannot manage the coal fire as he used to, and so the news of a changeover is greeted with a sense of relief by everyone. Praise the Lord for another breakthrough in answer to prayer.

27 September 2000 Dad's third visit to the Day Centre went fairly well – no complaints from either side. So far – so good!

29 September 2000 Dad rang to say that 'Aunty Joyce has been staying over and she's driving me mad! I can't do anything right for her – the tea is too hot or too cold. She doesn't want jam sandwiches as she's not hungry. She keeps hiding from me and going out into the middle of the road where she can get run over by the traffic!' I assured him that as Aunty Joyce was housebound suffering the effects of her stroke last year that she could not have been at his flat but instead he'd been having a vivid dream and that he wasn't to worry as Ken and Gaynor were looking after her. I suggested he take a little trip on the bus or go out for a walk in the fresh air to clear his head. He said, 'That's a good idea, Shirl – I think I will' and off he went. After all this time, I have learned to think of Dad as a little 'homing pigeon' because, in spite of the dementia, he always manages to come back to his own flat after being out for some time. Thank You again Lord!

4 October 2000 Dad's fourth visit to the Day Care Unit for assessment of suitability for regular attendance at the Centre. He appears to be adapting quite well to these once a week visits, but we'll have to see what his reaction is to the possibility of several visits per week as indicated by Bethan. Bethan feels that the Centre will probably offer Dad two days at first which will hopefully benefit Dad by giving his week more of a focus. I live in hope.

CHAPTER 20

More Meetings

5 October 2000 Delyth Hughes, the Occupational Therapist, is due to visit today at 10am. Before the staff at the Day Unit can finalize their report regarding Dad, they have to find out how he manages in his own home environment – hence Delyth's visit. After several questions and discussions, Dad asked Delyth if she would like a cup of tea. This was ideal, as part of her report involved the exercise of 'Making a Hot Drink' by the patient. It was evident to Delyth that although Dad knew the mechanics of the exercise, he had lost the sequencing of events in which things had to be done. This caused her to have concerns, particularly in the realm of cooking. Delyth then asked Dad if he would like to have the 'Meals on Wheels' service. He replied with a definite 'No thank you' and that was the end of that conversation!

8 October 2000 Alwyn's mother and Dad came down for lunch and tea today. We played cards and, despite a few lapses in memory on Dad's part, we managed to have a few good games. It has to be said that some days are better than others and perhaps this was one of Dad's better days – Thank You Lord!

9 October 2000 Alwyn's birthday. Picked up some shopping for Dad, collected his pension, returned his washing, sorted out his 'pocket money'. Gareth Morris called today to advise that there was a meeting on Wednesday to discuss Dad's future visits to the Day Centre. I feel regretful that we didn't take time out to celebrate Al's birthday today. It seems as if everything and everyone else appears to get crowded out. Please, Lord, help me not to feel guilty about wanting to spend time alone. Thankfully Alwyn is very supportive and I find it a great source of comfort that he is coming along with me to the Prayer Meeting. It is here, amongst God's people and His presence that we 're-charge our batteries' and are given the strength to carry on in this very demanding role of caring.

11 October 2000 Multi-Discipline Team Meeting at 10.30am at the hospital. Present: Managers of the Unit, Occupational Therapist, Social Worker, Community Psychiatric Nurse, Alwyn and myself. Following Dad's weekly assessment sessions, it was decided that Dad could be offered a place at the Unit for three days per week providing, of course, that he would be in agreement. I was so relieved – this was so much better than we had hoped for, but it had to be something that Dad would be prepared to accept. I gave a quick prayer to my heavenly Father concerning the welfare of my earthly father and Dad was brought into the meeting for his decision on the matter. When Sian Davies, the overall Manager, explained the situation to Dad, he seemed quite keen on the idea and afterwards he was taken back to his activity session. I just cried with relief. Thank You Lord for the answer to prayer yet again!

13 October 2000 There was a phone call from Dad – he'd lost his bus pass again. It was nowhere to be found and after much searching we decided to make enquires about the issue of a new one. The matter will have to wait until Monday when the relevant department is open.

16 October 2000 Long awaited repairs done to the flat by the Council. Dad went to get some more photographs for his replacement bus pass. Alwyn and I took him to the office to get a new pass and he caught the bus home.

17 October 2000 Called in to see Dad after our 'Young at Heart' service and reminded him that we would not be at home tomorrow as Alwyn was taking me out for the day to celebrate my birthday. He appeared very pleased that I had reminded him as he said he would have worried himself to death if he couldn't get an answer on the telephone! I said I would ring him in the morning again before we went out just to put his mind at rest. We left his flat and took Alwyn's mother home. Eventually we came back to our own home to 'unwind' by relaxing in a nice warm bath!

CHAPTER 21

Soup on the Stove

18 October 2000 I rang Dad at nine o'clock this morning but there was no answer – he'd more than likely gone shopping and I purposed to ring him again this evening. Al and I then set off on our quiet day out together. It did us both good to 'get away from it all' even if just for a day, as it is so important to do something which means quality time spent together as husband and wife. It is also very important to bear in mind that in order to deal with the strains of caring for a loved one, the carer also has to have 'time out' to just do whatever he or she enjoys on their own without having to feel guilty about it!

The phone rang at 7pm and the peace was shattered! Dad's neighbour rang to say that the smoke detectors in Dad's flat were making an awful noise and thick black smoke was filling the living room, kitchen and hallway and that the front door was ajar. There was no sign of Dad but there was a note left on the table. He'd put soup in a saucepan, left the electric cooker on and tried to make his way on the bus up to the Day Centre. Fortunately, on this occasion, he had left the front door ajar, otherwise Mr Morgan, Dad's neighbour, wouldn't have been able to go in and switch the cooker off and open the windows to let some of the smoke out. I thanked Mr Morgan and told him that we would be up to sort things out at once. When we arrived, we were met with such a mess. There was obvious evidence to show that Dad had been out for some time as there was a cold cup of tea on the table along with some stale jam sandwiches. The young lady from the upstairs flat came down and asked if she could have a chat with us. Having secured Dad's front door, Alwyn and I dutifully followed Megan through the garden gate and around to her front door. We all went into her flat and were offered a cup of tea. Megan and her partner, Dafydd, told us that this was not the first time that something like this had happened, and that also in the early hours of the morning they were awakened very often to the sound of Dad chopping sticks for the fire. Also Dad had been seen wandering around the streets very late in the night and, sometimes, in the region of two o'clock in the morning. I explained Dad's medical condition to the young couple (who have two small children) and advised them that the overall objective was to keep Dad in his own home environment for as long as possible providing, of course, that he was not a danger to himself or others. Obviously, this incident was very close to meeting this criteria for committing Dad to a full-time residential care situation. I then encouraged Megan and Dafydd to bring their concerns to the Social Services Department as I, too, intended to bring this matter to their attention first thing in the morning. Whilst we were discussing this matter upstairs, we heard Dad's front door slamming – he had come home! We went down only to find him on the phone trying to ring us. I asked him if he was alright and he said he'd been up the valley looking for the Day Centre. He said he went to the original Day Centre but there was no-one about. He then tried looking elsewhere but he couldn't find the new one and then someone sent him home. I explained the seriousness of what had happened in his absence and he refused to believe he left the cooker on or left the door ajar – 'If I don't move from this chair!' Poor Dad. His condition is becoming progressively worse. He then threatened to cut his throat with a razor because he was so depressed. I talked him out of that and told him that I loved him and if he did something like that, where would that leave me? I rang Derek for some support – he wasn't at home and I left a message with my niece. I reassured Dad of the right day and time and made him supper. Dad then apologized for all the trouble that had been caused, but I could detect that he was still unconvinced that it was all down to his actions as the words, 'It wasn't me!' kept cropping up all the time. Alwyn and I came home feeling emotionally drained but thankful to the Lord that the outcome was not worse. Happy Birthday Shirl!

19 October 2000 7.30am   I rang Dad to see how he was this morning and to remind him that it was 'Day Centre Day' today. He appeared to be unaffected by the mini-crisis last night and said he hoped the driver wouldn't be long before picking him up!

8.30am – I rang Social Services and spoke to Lynfa Jones in Gareth Morris's absence and told her of the events of yesterday evening. As I was relating the details, a feeling similar to that of grief overcame me and I asked Lynfa if she would explain the saga to those in charge at the Day Centre as I didn't feel able to repeat the same story again. Lynfa was very sympathetic and said she would let the relevant people know what had happened and not for me to worry.

9.30am – The Area Housing Manager rang me to enquire about Dad's condition as he had received a phone call from the couple in the upstairs flat. I briefed him on the situation and advised him to ring Dad's social worker for the full picture.

9.40am – Bethan rang to say that she'd been told about the recent events and thought that now was the time to introduce Meals on Wheels. I explained that Alwyn had immobilised the cooker so that there was no danger of Dad leaving it on again and agreed that the best course of action would be to have a hot meal delivered on the days that Dad was not attending Day Centre i.e. Monday, Wednesday and Saturday. This routine is to be implemented with effect from Monday.

CHAPTER 22

'Closer Than A Brother'

20 October 2000 In view of the recent incident, it has become more of a priority to get Dad's central heating converted in order to keep him in his own home. Bethan explained Dad's situation to Mr Owen, the Area Housing Manager, and asked if he could possibly speak to the Council Authority to bring some pressure to bear on getting the work done quickly. He agreed to do his best and was satisfied that everything possible was being done in order to keep Dad safe in his flat and also the people in the upstairs flat. I still feel uneasy about the fact that Dad is living on his own but the reply I keep getting is that, although Dad's medical condition is deteriorating, he is still in a position to make conscious decisions as to what he wants to do and where he wants to live. Therefore, under the present Mental Health Act, no-one can force Dad into doing anything against his will and his wishes must be respected. (I was once told that under the present law he has the 'perfect right to live in squalor' if he wants to and there is nothing anyone can do about it!). Today is Friday and so we plod on regardless doing the usual visitation of Alwyn's mother and Dad before finally getting home and 'crashing out'. I wonder if my brother will ring tonight? My heart cries out for him to help me bear some of the burden – but to no avail! The phone is silent. I know he can't do much by way of physical help but I long for the emotional help and support that only a sibling can give. However, it is a long time coming but I do not despair altogether for I am reminded that, 'There is a friend that sticketh closer than a brother' (Proverbs 18:24) and He more than makes up for any sense of loss that I may be feeling. Thank You

Lord. Another verse of scripture which brings me comfort is that, even if I were all alone in this experience and felt isolated, there is One that I could always turn to – '. . . for he hath said, I will never leave thee nor forsake thee. So that we may boldly say, the Lord is my helper, and I will not fear what man shall do unto me' (Hebrews 13:5-6).

23 October 2000 Alwyn and I made sure that we were at Dad's earlier today so that we could be there when the dinner lady called with Dad's first meal from the Meals on Wheels Services. I explained Dad's condition to the lady and she had already been briefed by Bethan. We arranged payment in advance for the week and it was understood that if Dad was not at home when the dinner lady called then the likelihood was that he would have his lunch out whilst shopping. (That was the theory – however it was yet to be tested in practice). We deliberately did not mention the words 'Meals on Wheels' as Dad has always resisted quite adamantly from the onset of his illness that he did not wish to have these services provided. Instead, I made out a notice which read: 'A hot lunch, similar to those provided at the Day Centre, will be delivered on Monday, Wednesday and Saturday'. This notice was duly posted on the wall near to the place where Dad sits by the table. He has said that he enjoys the meals at the Day Centre and so, hopefully, he will accept this new change to his routine without too much resistance. It is understandable that Dad does not wish to have more control taken from him by having his meals provided, but I assured him that no one was saying that he could not manage to cook for himself, but that because he sometimes gets forgetful to turn the stove off, it is safer to do things this way. He said, 'I suppose so!' but, knowing Dad as well as I do, I could detect a sense of inevitability in him. Is his illness now starting to sink in with him I wonder? Poor Dad.

25 October 2000 This evening, Alwyn and I were invited to our first 'Carers' Evening' which proved to be very helpful and informative. I jotted down a few rough notes with the intention of passing on the information learned to a few friends. (Please see Appendix 1).

28 October 2000 Dad rang at 2.15am – he thought it was the afternoon. When I explained that it was dark outside and that it was the early hours of the morning, he blamed the Government yet again for changing the clocks (this has become the principal reasoning behind Dad's way of thinking and the main excuse for getting the time wrong!). However, after about twenty minutes of reassuring him, he seemed to give in reluctantly to what I was saying and apologized for disturbing me.

31 October 2000 I rang Dad at 7.30am to remind him it was 'Day Centre Day' today – Tuesday – but he said he had some shopping to do! I suggested that he'd have some time to go shopping after he'd come home from the Centre. However, he misunderstood what I had said and consequently missed the volunteer driver. The manager at the Centre rang to inform me that Dad was not at home when the driver called and that it was their policy to make the relatives aware of 'the client's absence'. I explained to Sian that he'd probably gone shopping and that I would ring her as soon as I had made contact with Dad. At about 11am, the driver thought he'd go back to Dad's flat in the event that he'd come home. On arrival, there was Dad – back from his un-scheduled shopping trip and ready to go to the Day Centre!

2 November 2000 As agreed, I rang Dad at 7.30am to remind him that it was 'Day Centre Day' today – Thursday. Hopefully, he would stay in this morning to be picked up as arranged and that we would not have a repetition of Tuesday's saga! I told Dad I would ring him again after he had come home from the Centre to let him know how Josh's appointment went at the hospital. At this juncture, Dad still recognizes Josh (his great-grandson) and takes a keen interest in his well-being. He is always asking how Josh and Kiara (his great grand-daughter) are progressing. It seems as if he feels unthreatened by children and appears quite relaxed with them. Of course, the children take Granddad George at face value and it is good to see them together. Thank You Lord that the children are Your gifts to us. Help us to treasure them and to treat them, too, with the respect that they deserve as well as Dad.

CHAPTER 23

Fireworks

3 November 2000 Usual 7.30am reminder call to Dad. Collect 'Santa Tour' tickets, deliver Dad's shopping and washing to his flat, visitation of the sick and elderly, 'do the rounds' i.e. Alwyn's mother and Dad. Back home about 8.30pm!

4 November 2000 Day off! Michael and Toni took the children up to Dad's today and he was delighted to see them. Dad rang to say that he had lost his bus pass – again – and that he had reported it to the Bus Depot. I said that as it was Saturday, there was no-one available to issue him with a replacement pass until after the weekend i.e. on Monday. He became very moody to think that the matter could not be resolved before then. However, I did manage to persuade him in the end that it would be a wasted journey if he went down to Pontypridd because no-one would be in the office on the weekend. I still had a lingering feeling though that he didn't quite believe me!

7.30pm phone call from Dad's new Home Care lady. She advised me that she'd knocked Dad's door and rung the doorbell but that there was no response from inside the flat. She looked through the letter-box and saw Dad's walking stick and coat hanging up on the rack in the passage. The television and lights were on but no-one was responding from within, despite her loud calls. Obviously concerned, she rang me to let me know the situation and I said that the children had been up earlier and perhaps he had fallen asleep because he was tired. I said I would continue to ring him every quarter of an hour and if there was no answer, then I would look into the matter further. However, she offered to return to his flat at

10.30pm to check in on him on her way home from her evening out. I thanked her very much and she said she'd ring me later. Ring . . . Ring . . . Ring . . . Ring . . . Ring . . . still no answer! As I said before, when Dad goes out he's like a homing pigeon and, even though it was getting late, at this point I wasn't unduly worried and thought he was having some difficulty getting a bus back. That is not to say that I was entirely free of worry because there is always a niggling doubt as to 'What if something has happened to him?' However, when Dad's Carer rang to ask if we'd been in touch with Dad because she still couldn't get an answer, the panic bells started to ring just a little bit louder! I said that I'd been ringing all evening and if he was there he would surely have heard the phone ringing and so I concluded that he must have gone out and hadn't come home yet. He sometimes went out leaving the television and lights on and didn't always use his walking stick – and as for his coat still being on the rack – he had several from which he could choose to wear. I thanked the Carer very much for her concern and said that Alwyn and I would be up shortly to sort things out. We drove through Pontypridd and Porth looking out for Dad as we went but he was nowhere to be seen. The bus stops were void of anyone waiting and all seemed very eerie even though there were one or two late fireworks cascading through the blackness of the sky. We eagerly looked at every taxi that we saw passing to see whether Dad was occupying one of their seats, but they seemed to be full of late night bonfire party-goers wending their way home. Where, oh where is Dad? We continued our journey up Cymmer hill towards Trebanog still looking for any sign of Dad. We had been told on more than one occasion that he would attempt to walk home from Porth if there were no buses running so, if we couldn't find him now, we would have to go to his flat to see if he'd returned whilst we were out on our search.

Eventually, after an agonizing and fruitless search, we arrived at Dad's flat at 1.45am. On opening the door and shouting our usual greeting, we were met with the words, 'You're on the ball, Shirl, I've only just got up!' There was Dad, sitting in the kitchen with a cup of tea and a piece of toast having his breakfast. I cannot begin to describe the sense of relief and thanks to the Lord I felt in my heart at that particular moment. That is something that can only be understood by someone who has been in a similar situation. Mingled with my relief was a tinge of anger because of all the upset that had been caused throughout the evening. However, it must always be borne in mind that it is the illness and not the fault of the sufferer which has brought about these kinds of situations. It can be very easy to make the mistake of blaming the sufferer in such cases. It appeared that Dad had fallen asleep in front of the television and his hearing aid was in the 'off' position. Consequently he did not hear the telephone ringing throughout the evening or hear the Carer calling – 'If I don't move from this chair!' When I explained what had taken place he said he 'didn't know what all the fuss was about'. We settled him and advised him that we were going home to bed now that we knew he was safe and sound and I said I would ring him in the morning. Alwyn left first and went to the car whilst I closed Dad's front door. I stood there for some time waiting and then I heard Dad crying (whether in prayer or to himself I do not know) 'Oh God, what have I done to deserve this – I don't know what is happening to me. I may as well throw myself in the river now and have done with it all.' I felt numb – what was I to do now? I knew that part of me wanted to go back inside and console him but another part of me was in favour of going home because if I went back into the flat, I knew that I too would break down in front of Dad. That wouldn't do any good for either Dad or myself and so, although it was a very hard decision to make, I resolved to go home – but not before praying for the Lord to look after Dad for me! Perhaps I shouldn't have said 'Day Off' at the beginning of today's entry after all! Never mind – the Lord knows all about it and He is in control.

5 November 2000 Today is Sunday. After last night and the early hours of this morning's events, neither Alwyn nor I had much sleep. Alwyn rang Pastor to explain that we wouldn't be in church this morning but would be there this evening. We went up Dad's and made him lunch before going up to Alwyn's mother's. Dad seemed unaware of what had happened earlier and I thanked God that he was safe. He was looking forward to watching 'Songs of Praise' on the television and putting his feet up to watch the snooker later. Thank You Lord!

CHAPTER 24

Lenny

6 November 2000 Nia Edwards, the Community Occupational Therapist, rang this morning to enquire if there was any contact from the Council with regard to the proposed conversion of Dad's central heating system. When I replied that we hadn't heard anything, Nia advised us to ring her by the end of this month if there still hadn't been any progress. We called to see Dad, as usual, after picking up his pension and took him some shopping. When it came to sorting out his weekly allowance or 'pocket money' I had to re-explain the fact that we were now working in decimal currency and that the days of the halfpenny and the shilling piece were long since gone. Dad seemed to be unconvinced and wanted to have the last word as it were, and wouldn't budge from the fixed ideas that he had regarding the currency being used today. However, I managed to divert his attention onto something else and it seemed to work! Poor Dad! I'm so glad that he was willing earlier on to allow me to take over his financial dealings as he truly would be in a mess by now. (According to the note he wrote on my birthday card, he said that he thanked God every day for having 'such a brainy daughter', for if it wasn't for me, he wrote, he would be 'up to his neck in debt or in jail by now'). I don't know about the 'brainy' bit but I, too, thank God for giving me the opportunity to learn a little more patience and forbearance in every situation that we have encountered together as a family. It bears repeating time and time again that in all things God is working together for good to those who love Him and are the called according to His purpose (Romans 8:28).

7 November 2000 Reminder phone call to Dad at 7.30am to let him know that it is 'Day Centre Day' today. He thought it was the evening and said that it was too late to go now. I gently reassured him that it really was the morning and suggested that he was to get ready by 8.30am as the volunteer driver would be there in an hour's time to pick him up. Dad mumbled his annoyance at the Government for 'messing around with the clocks again' and reluctantly believed me that it was the morning after all. I said I would ring him later on when he came home. Meanwhile, Alwyn and I had to take our beloved cat 'Lenny' to the vet. When I told Dad that Lenny had been experiencing a bout of coughing and sneezing he said, 'Oh, I do hope the vet will be able to do something for her – I'll also send up a prayer for her, because I believe in prayer you know!' It didn't surprise me that Dad believed in the power of prayer but it did take me by surprise at the speed with which he latched onto the plight of a sick animal and showed such passionate concern.

It turned out that Lenny's blood results were favourable and that there was no apparent disfunction of her kidneys. She was given an antibiotic injection and we were told to bring her back to the vet again on Friday. When Dad heard the news, again he was very sympathetic and voiced his hopes that everything would be alright. I must confess that, although Dad has been fond of animals in the past, he has never shown such a degree of concern before. Perhaps this is one of the side effects of his complaint. For, to my amateur way of thinking, perhaps Dad can identify with a poor creature that is sick and cannot bring people to the understanding of what they are really feeling and to explain what is wrong. Who knows?

9 November 2000 Reminder call to Dad at 7.30am as described above. However, before calling Dad I pressed the 1471 number to see who had called last. At this point it must be explained that Alwyn and I have been receiving several phone calls in the early hours of the morning and they were always from Dad. These calls were always to tell us some insignificant piece of news (insignificant to us, but obviously not to Dad) and we would gently explain to him that it was the early hours of the morning and there was no urgent need for us to have that piece of information there and then. After establishing the fact that there was no emergency to deal with, I tried to explain that it was time for everyone to go back to bed and that I would ring him at 7.30am as agreed. It has become more obvious that this information is just not sinking in as Dad continues to ring at odd hours. Therefore, Alwyn and I agreed that, in order to get some sleep, we would have to switch off the main house telephones and put the mobile phone on standby from 9.30pm every night. The mobile phone number had been given to the Day Centre Staff, Social Services, Home Care Staff and the upstairs neighbours so that, should there be a genuine emergency at any time, then we would be contacted accordingly. Obviously, this is not an ideal situation but it is the only solution we could come up with in order for us to have some quality sleep to enable us to deal with the everyday demands that caring for someone with vascular dementia brings.

10 November 2000 Reminder call to Dad at 7.30am. Today we take Lenny back to the vet for a check-up and I reminded Dad that we would let him know what happened as soon as he came home from the Centre. As it happened, Lenny was given a booster injection and all went well, much to everyone's relief. We called in to see Dad as usual and the flat was noticeably cold. Dad was having difficulty lighting the fire and he had been putting all sorts of things in the grate to try and get the fire started e.g. plastic milk bottle, sugar, dried milk and even a plastic spanner from the garden strimmer! Once again, Alwyn and I cleaned the whole grate out from scratch. Throughout this exercise, Dad was quite keen on letting us know that he had 'emptied the ashes from underneath' and that 'there was a nice fire there this morning'. It seems strange that whenever we go up to the flat, 'the fire has just gone out!' It worries me that Dad cannot manage to keep the fire going – his hands are showing signs of being too near the fire when he eventually does manage to light it. I keep ringing to find out when something definite is going to be done about the changeover but to no avail.

CHAPTER 25

Another Prayer Answered

12 November 2000 Today is Sunday and Dad rang at 9am to say that he'd had his wallet stolen! He was in a bit of a state but I managed to calm him enough for him to explain what had happened. He said that he'd put his wallet in the inside pocket of his jacket before going to bed last night. However, in the morning it had gone and Dad was vehemently accusing the Home Care workers of stealing it. I told him to look carefully in all his pockets and in the wardrobe and anywhere else that he may have put his wallet for safe-keeping and that I would ring him later to see if he had found it. Before we went to church, I rang Dad to see if he had managed to find the 'missing' wallet. He was very subdued and said that there was no sign of it anywhere, despite a thorough search. I reassured him that we would be up after the service to help him to look for it. I also reminded him that he was due to come down to us today for lunch and tea along with Alwyn's mother. He appeared happy at that prospect and so we left for church, praying for the wallet to come to light and that the matter would soon be resolved. On entering the church, I was visibly upset at the way Dad's behaviour was changing and becoming aggressive to the point of being nasty with me on the phone. I tried to put the incident behind me but, although I had prayed about the matter, it was evident that I hadn't turned the situation completely over into the Lord's hands or else I wouldn't have become quite so upset. However, on learning about the latest incident, my church family prayed for us and committed the issue to the Lord in prayer and I started to feel a lot better. It did help to speak to our friend, Debby, about things as she understood exactly how I felt as she had been in the identical position to us and so could empathize in a deeper way. Thank You Lord for our church family and the source of comfort they bring us because we are one in Christ Jesus.

When we arrived at Dad's flat, we searched the places that Dad had said he had looked but to no avail. However, when Alwyn looked at the biscuit tin that Dad keeps all his 'bits and pieces' in, on removing the lid, there was Dad's 'missing', presumed stolen wallet on the top of the contents! Praise the Lord for answered prayer yet again! Dad was overjoyed at the find but adamantly denied putting it there – 'It wasn't me' and swore with the added oath, 'If I don't move from this chair!' It must be very frustrating for Dad to have such an awful short-term memory and yet his long-term memory is excellent to the degree of remembering even the minutest of details. It seems that, in order for us to believe him, Dad must invoke some serious calamity to befall him to highlight the sincerity of what he is saying. Of course there is such a strong need for him to be believed because of the shortness of his memory (from one hour to the next in some instances). At times like these, I find it best just to reassure him that we all tend to get a bit confused at times and just leave it at that.

On arrival at our house, Dad thought that we had moved again as 'this kitchen seems to be a bit bigger than the last one'. I said that he'd been here before but that he'd probably forgotten, and so we proceeded to play our game of cards. Dad seems a little more confused today but I put it down to the upset he'd experienced earlier in the day with the wallet incident. The rest of the day proved uneventful and Alwyn took our visitors home after dropping me off at the church for the evening service.

13 November 2000 Dad rang at 6.30am to complain that the driver hadn't turned up to take him to the Day Centre! He said that he'd been out by the garden gate waiting for him for over two hours in the freezing cold. I explained that if he looked on the wall-chart that I had made for him (timetable) there was no Day Centre on Mondays but instead, the dinner lady would be calling with his hot meal. He also said that he was having great difficulty in lighting the fire. I asked him if he'd had breakfast, to which he replied, 'Oh I had my toast ages ago!'

I suggested he made himself a hot cup of tea to warm him up and advised him that Alwyn and I would come up shortly to see to his fire. We arrived after Dad had had his lunch and he seemed a bit more settled but he hadn't gone to Porth shopping. We sorted the fire out, played cards and made sandwiches for tea. Dad seemed alright and we left about seven o'clock advising him that the evening Carer would be with him soon to supervise his medication. I also told him that 'Coronation Street' would be on TV soon as it was Monday night. Before leaving, I set out Dad's clean clothes on the spare bed as usual and told him that I would ring him in the morning to remind him that it was 'Day Centre Day'.

9.15pm – We had a phone call from the upstairs neighbours, Megan and Dafydd to say that there was a very loud noise coming from Dad's flat. The noise was described as that of a washing machine or tumble drier which had a problem with the motor (like a rumbling noise) and also there was the sound of running water from about 7.30pm and it had woken their little boy. Dafydd went downstairs to see what was going on and Dad said he had been to bed and was now getting ready for work and was in the middle of changing his clothes. The banging/rumbling noise turned out to be the hot water tank overheating due to the fact that the fire was drawing up fiercely. I advised Dad to draw off the water by having a bath but he refused saying he couldn't be bothered and that he was having an 'awful job' putting his trousers on. I told him to turn the dial on the side of the Parkray towards the kitchen and he asked, 'What dial?' I gently explained as I've done countless times before that the dial was to control the flow of air to the fire and that, by turning it towards the kitchen, the fire would stop drawing so fiercely and the noise would stop. He said he would have a look and he put the receiver on the table. Unknown to him, I could hear him moaning and grumbling and wishing that people would 'mind their own business' and saying 'Haven't they got better things to do than check up on me?' He came back to the phone and said that he'd turned the dial as I'd asked. When I told Dad that it was still Monday, he got very upset and said, 'How can it be? You are trying to confuse me – I'll end up in the nuthouse if this carries on!' I gently went through the day's events and what we had done, but he insisted point-blank that 'that was yesterday' and wasn't in any sort of mood to be persuaded otherwise. So I said, 'Well, Dad, you are going to have a very long wait for the driver to take you to the Day Centre.' By this time it was 10pm and he said, 'If he doesn't come to pick me up this morning – I'm not going again as I'm getting worse not better since going up there. I'll end up in the river or do something stupid to myself if this carries on!' Again I tried to reassure him and told him I would ring him in the morning at 7.30am. He then accused me of doing a very good job of confusing him and I told him to ring Derek if he didn't believe what I was saying. Dad said, 'If I tell Derek what you are telling me, he'll think that you've gone round the bend!'

14 November 2000 I rang Dad at 7.30am as agreed. He said that no-one had come to pick him up yesterday and he wasn't going 'to that place' again because 'they've got no system!' Once again I told him that the driver was due to pick him up between 8.30am and 9am and that he would be there shortly after the morning Carer had been to supervise his medication. He said, 'If no-one comes soon – I'm going out!'

CHAPTER 26

The 'Sally Army'

15 November 2000 As Dad was in such an aggressive mood yesterday, I thought it best to leave him to cool down a bit as there was just no reasoning with him. He was adamant that no-one came to fetch him and that is why he went shopping. It's getting more and more difficult to reason with him and it's causing quite a strain. I rang the Community Psychiatric Nurse and explained to her that I don't want to end up in an argument situation every time that Dad comes on the phone insisting that 'they've let me down again with the driver!' If I end up agreeing with him, I feel I've given up on him and that, possibly deep down, Dad's only been going to the Day Centre to keep me happy, but really it may be that he just wants to be on his own. The Nurse said that Dad was settling into the Day Centre routine OK and that there was no hint of any resistance to attending the Unit – in fact I was reassured that he was the 'life and soul' of the place and that he thrived on the company of others!

16 November 2000 Nothing unusual to report today! I rang Dad (who seemed to be in a better frame of mind today) to remind him that Alwyn and I would be picking him up after Day Centre tomorrow to take him and Alwyn's mother to the specially arranged meeting at our church. At this meeting, our pastor had invited the Salvation Army Band to provide the music for the 'Moody and Sankey' presentation evening. We thought Dad would be very interested in this service because of his childhood connections with the 'Sally Army'. Sure enough, Dad was very enthusiastic about going to the meeting and he began to relate tales about 'the old days'. I patiently listened (although I'd heard these stories many times before, I feel that if they are important enough for Dad to tell me, then I should show him the courtesy of hearing him out) and then said that I would ring him in the morning at 7.30am as we'd agreed to remind him that it was 'Day Centre Day'.

17 November 2000 As promised, I rang Dad with the usual prompt and he seemed to have his bearings, as it were, this morning, as he said he was looking forward to going to see the Salvation Army Band tonight. Day Centre went without incident and all seemed fine when we picked Dad up this evening. However, Dad hadn't changed his shirt for about a week and it was looking a bit the worse for wear. When I suggested that he should change his clothes, he became quite nasty. He also smelled of urine which was quite embarrassing, but he refused point-blank to change. (Previously, when I've noticed that Dad has put his trousers to dry in the airing cupboard amongst the clean clothes, I've gently asked him to put any 'wet' trousers/underpants in the bath so that I could find them easily and wash them accordingly. He raised no objection to this suggestion). Today, however, I guess he may have been over-eager to go to the meeting and didn't want to be delayed by the time it would have taken him to change. So, off we went and had a very enjoyable evening.

Dad was thrilled to bits at the children singing and with the Band playing all the old familiar hymns of long ago. How they must have conjured up even more memories of days gone by when he, as a young lad, went to the 'Sally Army Sunday School' and to the other services in the week. As I sat next to Dad, it was obvious that he couldn't read all the words on the hymnsheet but nonetheless, his memory served him well on this occasion as he sang with gusto the wonderful words 'What a Friend we have in Jesus, all our sins and griefs to bear, what a privilege to carry everything to God in prayer...' and I could tell, he really meant what he was singing!

Thank You Lord. After the service, we all had refreshments and then took Dad back to his empty, lonely flat. What a contrast. How I wish that Dad would agree to live in a residential home. There he would have company whenever he wanted to and also have his own privacy likewise. I continue to pray to that end.

19 November 2000 Today is Sunday and Alwyn and I took Dad his lunch. I showed Dad, once again, how to use the microwave cooker, but he didn't appear to be all that interested. He seemed to be in a strange mood, as if he had only just woken up and didn't quite know where he was. I reminded him that it was Sunday and that my mother-in-law was expecting Alwyn and myself to visit her for lunch and that she was expecting us there by 1pm. He said he didn't want us to be late and that it was 'very nice of you to come up to see to my dinner for me'. We left Dad eating his meal but I had a gnawing kind of feeling in my stomach and felt uneasy about leaving him on his own. The weekends tend to be the worse time for Dad, especially when there are no buses running until late afternoon. It's as if Dad craves for attention or company, but he still refuses to give up his independent way of life and so, in a way, is his own worst enemy. I just keep praying that the Lord will make a way where, seemingly at the moment, there is no way.

CHAPTER 27

Time and The Silent Killer

24 November 2000 I rang Dad for the usual reminder prompt for the Day Centre visit. There was no answer. 7.40am – no answer. 7.50am – no answer. 8.00am – no answer. 8.10am – Dad answered! He'd been down to Porth shopping but couldn't get a bus back until now! According to Dad the bus driver told him there were at least seventeen buses off the road and that he would be quicker walking home (some distance of two miles all uphill). When I told him that the volunteer driver would be there in twenty minutes or so to pick him up and take him to the Day Centre, Dad's reply was, 'What? At this time of night? If they think I'm going all the way up there at this time of night – they've got another thing coming! I'm too tired anyway – I'm going to bed!' On assuring Dad that it was the morning and not the night, he said, 'Well I don't see how it can be! There are only 24 hours in a day, so why do they keep messing about with the clocks all the time for? I don't know whether I'm coming or going – and I'm not on my own either – I've heard a lot of people talking and they say the same thing as me! The Government should leave the clocks alone.' Not wanting to enter into the same debate again, I just re-affirmed the correct time of day and advised Dad that I would ring him later this afternoon when Day Centre was over and then rang off.

Dad rang at 8.30am and said quite excitedly, 'What do you think, Shirl? That driver just came to pick me up for Day Centre and asked me if I was ready to go! I soon told him – fancy coming around at this time of night to go to a Day Centre. He would insist on telling me that it was the morning but I told him not to be so dull and to go away as I was too tired and wanted to go to bed!' I asked Dad where the driver was now and Dad said that he had 'sent him packing'. I just couldn't believe my ears. Here was Dad telling this kind volunteer driver to go away, and I had only just explained about ten minutes ago that it was indeed the morning and Dad had reluctantly agreed. However, it did prove to be a reluctant belief on his part due to the fact that he told the driver to go away as it wasn't the right time to go visiting the Day Centre! I just give up trying to explain sometimes and tend to lose patience in the end. I told Dad that he would be missing out on his lunch at the Centre today as a result of his actions and that he would have to fend for himself food-wise somehow until we came to visit him later.

The Staff at the Day Centre rang to say that Dad hadn't turned up this morning and I explained what had transpired earlier and apologized for Dad's behaviour towards the driver. Hannah said she understood and said that as long as Dad was OK then they would see him again on Tuesday.

On arrival at Dad's flat this evening, we were met with Dad fast asleep on the settee with his hat and overcoat on and the fire unlit. The flat was decidedly cold as a result, and at first, fear gripped my heart as I saw Dad curled in a heap. I bent over him and tentatively put my hand on his neck to see if there was a pulse. Please, Lord, let Dad be alright. With that, Dad stirred himself and began to sit up – he'd fallen into a deep sleep as he didn't hear us coming in, he said. When he was more awake I asked him why the fire wasn't lit. He said that he couldn't get it to light as he didn't have any sticks and he'd 'tried everything on it' but the fire still wouldn't light. I made him a hot cup of tea and then set about emptying the whole grate which was clogged up. I can't believe that Dad has used up all the firewood which we brought him not so very long ago. However, I did manage to find some off-cuts in the bottom of the cardboard box and so began the task of re-laying the grate. Soon, there was a lovely fire and both the room and the water began to get warm again. Once more I patiently explained how the Parkray worked and before I had finished my sentence, Dad was telling me how to do things! It seems as if he needs constant prompts in order for his skills to 'kick-in' as it were, and then there's no stopping him from giving all the instructions necessary in order to light the fire. However, there is a world of difference between the theory and the practical and, unfortunately, Dad has lost the art of sequence in this respect. It begs the question, though, 'What would have happened if for some reason Alwyn and I couldn't have made our visit to Dad tonight?' Hypothermia is a silent killer and a friend to the lonely. Please Lord, keep Dad safe.

CHAPTER 28

'Where Are The Children?'

25 November 2000 Today is Saturday – I wonder what this weekend will bring? It seems as if Dad is worse on the weekends. Perhaps because there is not so much interaction with other people or maybe he just feels more lonely on the weekends. One thing is sure, however, I must not beat myself with the 'big stick of guilt' where Dad is concerned on these two days of the week as it is vital that I keep a balance with looking after my husband's and grandchildren's needs as well as those of my own. The Meals on Wheels lady calls today and so I know that Dad will have a hot meal at lunchtime and I usually phone him to remind him to make a sandwich or 'Cuppa Soup' for later in the day. Meanwhile, I'm looking forward to an evening out to supper with some very dear friends with whom I lost touch quite some years ago.

26 November 2000 After this morning's service, Alwyn and I called up to see Dad and to give him his lunch as usual. However, on this occasion, lunch was to be a hastily thrown together affair! Dad had managed to render the microwave cooker inoperable (probably by putting a metal object in it or by leaving it on for too long). Of course, according to Dad, 'It wasn't me! I didn't do it. If I don't move from this chair!' Fortunately, Dad's cupboard was stocked with packets of 'Cuppa Soups' which proved to be very useful on this occasion. His lunch, therefore, consisted of a bowl of soup, two ham rolls and a packet of crisps followed by a cup of tea and chocolate cake. There was plenty of tinned fruit and evaporated milk in the fridge for tea, along with a variety of biscuits and cream crackers. I explained to Dad that my mother-in-law was expecting us for lunch at one o'clock as usual and that I would ring him this evening to see how he was. As we were leaving, Dad asked, 'Where are the children? Why aren't you taking them with you?' Quite puzzled by these questions, I replied with another question, 'What children, Dad?' to which he answered between mouthfuls of soup, 'Well your children of course – you left them with me when you went out this morning – they've been back and forth all day!'

'My children are grown up, Dad', I said, 'do you mean Josh and Kiara?' (My younger son's children). At this point, Dad became quite agitated and said, 'No! I know Josh – I'm talking about your children – where are they?'

When I explained that my children weren't small any more but that they had in fact grown up into adult young men, Dad seemed quite bewildered by that thought and he proceeded to look for them in the bedroom and in the kitchen. Unable to find them, he shrugged his shoulders and said, 'Well, I don't know where they've gone – they've been playing happily about the place until now – I thought that perhaps Alwyn had taken them for a walk over the mountain.' Poor Dad, he is so confused but rigid in his belief that he is right, and finds it very difficult to accept otherwise. In the end, I suggested that perhaps he'd fallen asleep earlier and had dreamed about the children playing in his home and then I comforted him with a hot cup of tea. I pray that these delusions will stop soon as it is quite upsetting to see the effect they are having on Dad. He seemed a bit more settled when we left, but I must admit, I didn't feel too comfortable leaving him in the flat on his own. Please Lord, will you befriend Dad as you have befriended me?

Alwyn's mother's phone rang at about 2.30pm – it was Dad. 'Will you come and fetch me and take me home? Ken can't take me up there as his car is in the garage for repair and Aunty Joyce isn't in. There are no buses running and if you can't take me home, then I'll have to walk all the way – that's all there is to it!' As it happened

Dad was already in his own flat but he was talking about 'the other Shrewsbury Avenue' which only exists in his own mind. I explained that he was phoning from his own home as we'd only left him having his lunch there not so long ago. He was adamant that he was going to walk home as he couldn't stay in 'this hole' any longer! As it was Sunday, the bus service wouldn't start until about 3pm and when I told Dad this he said that he would catch the bus home! When I said that it was Alwyn's mother's turn to be visited today and not his, he changed his attitude in that he agreed it was only fair that we should visit her as well because she was a widow, living on her own also in need of company. I said I would ring him later when we got home and there was no more talk of him 'walking home'.

As promised, I rang later in the evening to see how he was and he appeared to be fine, commenting on how he had enjoyed watching 'Songs of Praise' on the television. 'Goodnight Dad – I'll phone you in the morning OK? God bless.'

CHAPTER 29

The Strangers

27 November 2000 'Did you know who those strangers were in my flat last night, Shirl?' asked Dad quite nervously this morning as he rang me at 7.50am. 'They were whispering rumours and saying that Morfy was dead – do you remember Morfy, Shirley?' Before I could answer, Dad went on to say how cheeky these people were – even coming into his bedroom and sitting on his bed and whispering together in a huddle. He said that he couldn't rest and so went down to the house where Morfy lived but couldn't get an answer. It was raining heavily and the wind was keen (a 'lazy wind' as Dad called it, i.e. a wind that went through you rather than around you!) and as there was no answer at the house, Dad had assumed that these strangers' tales had to be true and that in fact Morfy had to be dead. He related that the only thing he could do in these circumstances was to make his way back to his flat in the pouring rain and write out a 'Notification Sheet' for the Registrar. 'I was soaked through,' Dad exclaimed. At this point, I interrupted Dad and asked if he was alright and had he changed his wet clothes and had a hot cup of tea. He said that his fire had gone out and that he couldn't get it to light. However, he had managed to take his wet clothes off 'somehow' and put some dry ones on with some difficulty before having a cup of tea. Poor Dad. This just cannot continue. I reassured him that we would be up in a short while to sort things out. I explained to him that Morfy (my mother's sister) had died about seven years ago, and that we had all gone as a family to the funeral. He said that he couldn't remember and he furrowed his brow and said, 'I don't recall that, Shirl – it's as if my mind has gone into the next world or somewhere!' He said that by the time he came back to the flat, the dustman had been and he was upset that he hadn't put his bin out for collection. When I told him that it wasn't 'bin day' until Wednesday, he was pleased that he hadn't missed the collection, but upset that he'd got the days of the week mixed up. After reassuring him that we would be up to see him shortly Dad said, 'Sorry to keep troubling you like this, Shirl – I don't know what I'd do without you!'

As it was now the last week in November, I was asked to ring Nia Edwards (the Community Occupational Therapist) to ask her whether there had been any news from the contractor with regard to the proposed conversion of Dad's central heating system. As there had been no contact at all, Nia rang the people concerned to see what was the latest position. On enquiring, Nia was told that a 'hiccough' had arisen in that the contractor appointed to the task had broken his ankle and, therefore, was unable to commence the work for some time. Apparently, if the work was to be given to another contractor it would mean that new cost estimates etc would need to be calculated and submitted to the Council and that exercise in itself would mean additional time consumption. Nia said that she would speak to the Area Housing Manager on Dad's behalf and press the urgency of the situation to him. Perhaps he could bring some authority to bear on the situation – but of course there could be 'no guarantees'. I thanked Nia for her help and said that I would contact her if there were any further developments. Meanwhile, I rang Menai Williams (the Community Psychiatric Nurse allocated to Dad's case whilst Bethan was on sick leave) and related to her my increasing concerns about Dad's safety and well-being. The fact that Dad was now acting on these 'delusions' or 'memory pop-ups' was of grave concern to me. Now he was subconsciously being forced to go out in adverse weather conditions and possibly contract pneumonia or collapse through sheer exhaustion at the attempt. At this point, I started to cry at the very thought of what I'd just said to Menai and immediately she said, 'I think we should have a review of Dad's situation with everyone concerned, Shirley. You are understandably upset and I feel we should have a get together and talk things over. Are you alright – is someone with you?' When I said that Alwyn was with me, Menai told me that she would contact the Social Services Department and try to arrange a meeting as soon as possible and would ring me back with the details. At last! I felt as if a burden had been lifted but still felt a gnawing sensation in the pit of my stomach. Then I prayed, 'Lord, please undertake for us as a family once more – Your Word says that You will never leave us nor forsake us, so I am confident that You will see us through this experience – come what may! Thank You. Amen.' Menai rang about a half hour later and said, 'If it's convenient with you and your husband, Shirley, the review will take place at 1pm at the Day Centre on Wednesday.' Without checking my diary or calendar, I said it was fine as I felt that this matter was far too important an issue to postpone. So, it was all agreed.

Alwyn and I arrived at Dad's and we were met with a rather forlorn-looking character who was fast asleep on the settee, blissfully unaware of his cold and grubby surroundings. Alwyn went to make the tea, when I started to rake out the cold, grey ashes from the grate. Dad stirred. 'Is that you Shirley? I'll make a cup of tea now – the kettle has only just boiled.' When there was a nice, big, safe fire and after a hot meal, I suggested to Dad that maybe I could make enquiries for him to visit the Day Centre every day instead of three days a week. 'What do you think, Dad?' I asked, 'would you like to be able to go every day if it could be arranged? Then you would know that every morning someone would be picking you up to take you out and perhaps you wouldn't get quite so confused about what day it was.' He agreed that it sounded a good idea and I said I'd try my best to find out if it was possible. Today is Monday – Prayer Meeting evening – once more, we've got plenty to thank the Lord for and to lay our burdens at His feet. Thank You Lord.

CHAPTER 30

The Review and The Response

29 November 2000 Review day. Everyone was there except Gareth Morris, Dad's social worker. I was disappointed at him not being there as he has been very supportive throughout this whole ordeal that we've been going through as a family. However, when the reason for his absence was recorded, I understood why it had been difficult for him to attend and so quickly began my task of concentrating on the matter in hand. Sitting on my left hand side was Menai, who was accompanied by Sian Davies, the Manager of the Day Centre. Next to Sian sat Hannah Griffiths, another Care Manager at the Unit. Hannah was flanked by one of the four assistants allocated to Dad's care whilst he visited the Centre and to her left sat Delyth Hughes, the Occupational Health Therapist. The circle was completed with Alwyn sitting between Delyth and myself. Before the review meeting started, I had broached the subject of the possibility of Dad being able to make daily visits to the Unit and that he was agreeable if it could be arranged. Menai officially started the meeting by saying how she had called it into being. It was on the basis of her concerns for Dad's welfare now that things were beginning to take on a new turn. She said that she was also concerned that I was becoming more and more distressed with coping with Dad, as was borne out by our telephone conversation on Monday. Sian then asked me what it was that I wanted to see happening for Dad. Sian was very pleased to have Dad to attend the Day Centre on a daily basis but, in her opinion, that wouldn't necessarily afford the peace of mind that I was craving for by way of Dad being looked after properly on a 24 hour basis. It would only serve as a 'stop-gap'. However, Sian advised that the option was open at the present time for a full-time residential care situation as there were just a few places available within the local area. Here I was faced with the stark reality. An opportunity was presenting itself whereby Dad could have all the necessary care (which he obviously needed and I could not provide) and I could be relieved of quite a lot of the pressure that comes with caring for a loved one whom you know is not going to get better – rather worse. Again, I turned to my faithful Friend in a silent prayer, asking for His guidance in the matter and seeking His reassurance. After what seemed an eternity (but actually only a minute or so) I said, 'I want whatever is best for Dad under the circumstances – I want to see him safe and well cared for all the time. If this means Dad having to go into a residential or nursing home, then so be it. One thing I ask is that you broach the subject with him, and not me, as I know from past experience that Dad will probably be against the idea. Perhaps he'll take it better coming from an "authority figure" than from me.' Alwyn put his arm around my shoulder to comfort me as by this time I was very upset. Sian said that from past experience she knew that this was an upsetting time for the relatives, but that we were not to look upon the situation as 'putting Dad into a Home' but rather that we were giving him the opportunity to live in a safer environment and allowing him to have a better quality of life. He would be able to have company or privacy whenever he wanted and have all his meals on a regular basis. This, in itself, would possibly help him to become more focused on the time of day etc giving him a better sense of orientation than he is experiencing now. Also the dangers of wandering about the streets at all hours and in all sorts of weather conditions would be greatly reduced. Although all these were very positive aspects and advantages, I was still plagued by a small element of inner guilt at the thought of Dad having to leave his home to go and live in another place. He would no longer be 'Master' in his own home – and how he loved to be 'his own boss'.

However, I had to ask the Lord to take that misplaced guilt away as I knew that for Dad to have more time with us on this earth, he would have to be taken care of in a manner that I could not provide – and that was that! After all, we would still be visiting him twice a week and I would still be arranging all his financial affairs and putting things in order for him. We would not be abandoning him, but rather giving him the freedom of a better way of living. Sian said to leave the matter with her and that she would have a word with Dad tomorrow about the prospect of having someone to look after him full-time and she would ring me to let me know how she got on. Through my tears, I thanked everyone in the meeting for their help and support and I shook each one of them by the hand before leaving for home.

30 November 2000 7.30am – I rang Dad to remind him it was 'Day Centre Day' today but did not give him any clue as to what was going to be discussed. I thought I would leave it to the professionals!

9.30am – Sian phoned to say that an opportunity had come for sheltered accommodation in the area and had asked Dad how he felt about the prospect of going to live in one of the homes where he could have all the care that he needed and deserved. She said that after a discussion with Dad, he was agreeable to the suggestion but wanted to talk it over with me first before committing himself to anything final. When Sian handed the phone over to Dad, I sounded really positive and asked him how he felt about the situation. He replied, 'What do you think, Shirl? It sounds good doesn't it? I think I'll give it a go!' You could have knocked me down with a feather! I quickly gathered my thoughts and said, 'Look, Dad, at the end of the day it is your decision. Personally, I feel it is a very good idea. If it was me, I would accept the offer but it is entirely up to you. I'm not telling you what to do and no-one should force you into doing something you don't want to do. Think it over today and we'll talk more about it when we come up tomorrow (Friday) OK?' With that, he said, 'OK love but I've got nothing to lose, so I think I'll give it a go anyway!'

Well, well – thank You Lord – here was prayer being answered on our behalf yet again. I really don't know how people manage without this Friend of mine. Sian came back on the phone after returning Dad to his activity group and said, 'Shirl, Dad came in this morning and he was really cold, his hands were covered in minor cuts and he had chafing behind his ear. So I took the opportunity as I was giving him a hot cup of tea and attending to "his wounds" of asking him his opinion of what he thought about the idea of someone being able to look after his needs like this every day and being able to live in warm, comfortable surroundings. He said, "Chance would be a fine thing!" When I said that it could happen for him because there were a few coveted places available and if he was agreeable, I could put his name forward for such a place – he actually beamed a smile from ear to ear! Of course he wanted to talk things over with you first because, "me and my daughter are very close and I want to know what she thinks about it." I felt I ought to strike whilst the iron was hot and so there we are. I'll send you a list of homes within the area which have places available, but obviously it's not up to me to recommend any one place in particular. You will need to make that decision as a family once you've asked all the necessary questions about the proposed home of your choice and had a look around at their facilities. Let me know how you get on, and if there is anything I can do to help – just let me know OK? 'Bye.'

Alwyn made us a nice hot cup of tea and I sipped mine slowly as the conversation I'd just had with Dad and Sian began to sink in.

CHAPTER 31

Added Grace and On A Mission

1 December 2000 Unfortunately Dad, once again, had not been at home when the volunteer driver had called to pick him up for the Day Centre. This was in spite of my reminder call at 7.30am. Never mind, it so happened that the driver went back later and picked Dad up so that he didn't miss out on his visit. These people are so kind – I thank God for them all.

Our conversation this evening at Dad's was quite positive. We discussed the benefits, not only for Dad but also for me as he agreed that I would have a 'lot less running about' to do if he were living in a residential home. Also his laundry would be taken care of so that would alleviate my load in more ways than one! This positive mood continued into the playing of cards with Dad seeming to win every game this evening as I recall.

Before leaving, I laid out Dad's clean clothes on the spare bed as usual and collected his bag of soiled washing – only this evening it seemed to weigh so much lighter! Goodnight Dad. God Bless!

4 December 2000 The list of residential/nursing homes had arrived by this time and Gareth was due to meet Alwyn and myself to sort out the necessary assessment forms. This was it. The meeting was scheduled for 10.30am at Dad's flat whilst Dad was at the Day Centre. However, Dad did not go with the driver this morning as there was an argument over the time of day (Dad insisted that it was 8.30pm and not 8.30am and, therefore, sent the driver away in no uncertain terms!). Therefore, when Alwyn and I turned up at the flat, we were surprised to see Dad, sitting down in 'the chair' having his supper! 'You're late, Shirl – was it raining when you came in?' After having painstakingly explained that it was the morning and not the evening, Dad trumped up, 'Well, I'm not going to the Day Centre at this time of night anyway and, in fact, I don't think I'll go somewhere else to live either! They'll shove me up on top of a mountain or somewhere in the back of beyond I expect, knowing my luck!' My heart sank. No amount of reasoning on my part would change his mind or cause him to see that no-one was going to 'shove him' anywhere he didn't want to go. He was defending his territory as best he could – and if that meant trying to manipulate me into feeling guilty – then he was doing a very good job! However, I prayed for help to deal with this situation and, true to His Word, the Lord gave me added grace and inner strength to be able to cope.

The doorbell rang – it was Gareth. I hurriedly went to the door to forewarn Gareth that Dad hadn't gone to the Day Centre because of the confusion over the times and also that Dad was very reluctant to move from his home. I tried very hard to hold back the burning tears and composed myself before re-entering the living room. Gareth stood in the doorway and Dad looked up from his chair to the very official-looking gentleman with a black leather briefcase and long dark overcoat. 'You haven't gone to the Day Centre this morning, Mr Dowling, how is that?' 'Well,' said Dad this time hesitantly, 'only a few minutes ago, I had to send the driver away. Fancy coming at this time to pick me up. I don't like to put anyone into trouble, but he's not very reliable you know – he comes just when he likes and expects me to go with him! There's just no system with the fellow!' Gareth didn't argue but just said in a loud clear voice – 'Never mind that for now, Mr Dowling, would you still like to go? If you do, I've got my car outside and I can take you if you like.' 'Oh yes please,' said Dad, 'that's very kind of you – I'll just put my coat on and I'll be with you.' Dad couldn't get to the coat hooks fast enough! 'Are you coming, Shirl?' asked Dad. I explained that Alwyn and I were going to do some cleaning and have his tea ready when he came home. Off Dad went with Gareth, with no trouble or grumbles at all – leaving Alwyn and myself staring at each other in disbelief of what we had just witnessed. Talk about 'Dr Jekyll and Mr Hyde'!

I rang Sian at the Day Centre and explained that Gareth was on his way with Dad. I briefed her on this morning's happenings and Dad's change of mind and Sian asked if Dad had made known his feelings to Gareth. When I said, through my tears, 'No,' Sian said, 'Good – leave it to me – I'll ring you back later. Don't worry!' How many times have I uttered those very same words to other people and now, someone was telling me. It was then that I was reminded of a verse in the Bible which says, 'Casting all your care upon Him for He careth for you' (1 Peter 5:7). Again I prayed to my faithful Friend and had a hot cup of tea to try and get myself more composed by the time Gareth came back.

After a short while, Sian rang to say that Gareth was on his way back after having a chat with Dad at the Centre. Sian said, 'Dad was as meek as a lamb, Shirl – he showed no aggression at all with us and when I told him that a place had become available for him he was very pleased. It's like this, Shirley, none of us likes the thought of giving up our home do we? So Dad was making his defence in the only way he knew how – by "pressing the right buttons" as far as you, his daughter, were concerned. By taking him out of the situation and bringing him up to the Day Centre, we were able to reason things out with him from a professional standpoint and help him to see what action would serve his interests best. So, don't worry, now Shirley, Dad is OK about it now – really. Gareth is on his way down, I'll speak to you again soon. 'Bye.'

Once again the Lord had intervened on our behalf. What a mix of emotions and questions came into being. The realization of what Sian had described regarding Dad 'pressing the right buttons' suddenly dawned on me – poor Dad, was he so desperate that he had to resort to emotional blackmail? He had no-one else to turn to for support in his struggle to maintain the little independence he enjoyed and now, was I turning against him in this fight? Was Dad just saying, 'Yes' to keep everyone happy but deep down, was his heart crying out, 'Treason'? Then I found myself being told by the still small inner voice not to feel guilty in any way, as what was going to happen was all in Dad's best interests and that everything would work out well in the end. That inner voice was echoed by my husband's audible voice which now confirmed what I was really beginning to feel. Until now, the prospect of Dad going into a home for the elderly and mentally infirm had somewhat paralysed me, but now, after today, I decided that if this was really going to come to pass, then we must make all the preparations as quickly and as painlessly as humanly possible with God's divine guidance.

Gareth arrived, we sorted out all the paperwork and set about the task of seriously looking through the list of homes in front of us. Sian said that we should choose two in case the first choice was not suitable after having viewed the premises etc and then we could fall back on the second choice. This procedure would have to be repeated until we came to a home which we felt was appropriate for Dad's needs. Then we would need to make an appointment to view and ask our many questions and take it from there. 'Brynteg' was our first choice as it was conveniently situated near the family and it would provide easy visiting access on a regular basis. However, when I rang to ask if there was a place available, it turned out that it was a Nursing Home rather than a Residential Home – and although Dad is suffering from vascular dementia, he is not at the last stage of the illness yet which requires the services of such a home as Brynteg. I thanked the Matron very much for her kindness in dealing with me and so, undeterred, and with another silent prayer, turned to our second choice – 'Seion'. This time, a gentleman answered when I rang. It was Mr Glyndwr Evans, one of the Directors at the Home. I explained the situation to him and asked if there were any rooms available. The reply was like music to my ears! 'Yes, Mrs Ashman, in fact there are two rooms available – one double and one single with effect from 8th December. Would you like to see them and speak to the Deputy Manager in charge of the care side of things?'

'Oh yes please,' I said, 'when would it be convenient for us to visit?' 'Any time that's convenient for you, Mrs Ashman, no need to make an official appointment – just drop in whenever it suits you.'

Despite the fact that an appointment wasn't necessary, I felt it only a courtesy on my part to let Mr Evans know that we would be there at 2.15pm. After a hasty lunch, Alwyn and I set out to see what was in store for us at Seion. We chose Seion also for convenience of visiting as it is literally only a stone's throw away from Alwyn's mother's home. However, time did not permit us to visit Mam today as we were on a mission and it had to be completed before Dad came home from Day Centre or he would have been coming into an empty flat with no tea ready!

Armed with Dad's personal file, I rang the doorbell of this wonderful, stone-built Welsh chapel which had been converted into a Home for the elderly. Ifan Price, one of the Carers, opened one half of the great wooden, outer secured doors and led us into the beautifully decorated hallway. Ifan then took us to meet Mr Evans and, as it happened, Alwyn knew him! Well, this was a good start, don't you think? Whilst the men chatted in general, I stood gazing at the surroundings. To think that these walls had once echoed with the sounds of people praising God! How humbled and privileged I felt at that moment to think that maybe this was God's choice for Dad. I prayed that it might be true! We were shown around the whole building and we were very impressed indeed. My initial response was, 'If the situation were reversed, would I like to come and live here?' and I had to say 'Yes, I would', in that it felt very comfortable and there was a pleasant atmosphere. I was particularly impressed by the absence of the smell of stale urine and rank body odour – indeed there was a very pleasant fragrance throughout the whole building. The file, which I had carried around with me on our guided tour, was bursting with questions and so I proceeded to 'interrogate' Heulwen Davies who, I must say, adopted a very helpful attitude throughout the whole of our visit.

Q. What medical cover is there in case of any emergencies at the Home?

A. A District Nurse calls several times a week and GP cover is also available when needed.

Q. What about visiting? Are there any set hours?

A. There are no restrictions – any time – day or night.

Q. What is the ratio of staff to residents?

A. There are four members of staff on duty at any given time. Care is provided 24 hours a day. The Home can accommodate up to 31 people.

Q. Have the residents access to local shops with staff accompaniment?

A. Yes. Also day trips/outings are planned fairly regularly.

Q. What about daily activities?

A. There is a timetable of weekly events on the notice board in the dining room. These activities include board games, cards, dominoes, quizzes etc. A fortnightly church service is held by the local pastor.

Q. What about furniture for the room?

A. All the basic furniture is provided such as a bed, wardrobe, dressing-table, two easy chairs, stool and small table. The residents provide their own TV/Radio.

Q. Is there access to a telephone?

A. Yes – via the main office at the front of the building.

Q. What about laundry facilities?

A. All the residents' laundry is done on the premises.

Following our 'Question and Answer Session', I apologized to Heulwen in case I had overstepped the mark by asking so many questions. I just felt the need to be so thorough because, after all, I was about to hand over the care of my father to complete strangers and I wanted to make sure that, if Dad was going to be accepted as a resident in Seion (or any other place for that matter) then I needed to find out as much information as I possibly could. Heulwen said that she was happy to answer any queries that I may have regarding the Home and assured me that she was glad that I was asking such questions as, in her view, it showed that I was really interested in Dad's well-being and was only doing what she herself would be doing if the circumstances were the other way around. Several times, Alwyn and I were asked if we wanted a cup of tea or coffee but, as time was at a premium, we had to refuse (much to my dismay I may add – as it is very rare that I refuse a cup of tea!!).

We left Seion, promising Mr Evans that we would get in touch with Gareth to let him know that we were happy to make this place Dad's new home. My heart was pounding at the prospect that very soon we could be visiting Dad in a whole new setting.

When we arrived at Dad's flat, I rang the Social Services Department and asked to speak to Gareth. Unfortunately, Gareth had gone home unwell and so I rang Sian at the Day Centre. I explained that we'd been up to view Seion and that we were very impressed by our visit but we were unable to contact Gareth with our decision. Sian advised me to ring Mr Evans and explain that Gareth was unavailable until tomorrow but would it be possible to reserve a place for Dad pending the completion of the paperwork. Mr Evans said that it would be alright and said that his colleague, Mr Llewellyn, would be in contact with Social Services tomorrow. Time for that cup of tea now I think!

Dad arrived home and we enjoyed our sandwiches and crisps together (and yes – another cup of tea!) followed by a short game of cards. There was no mention of Dad not wanting to move which I took as a good sign and so resigned myself to the thought that, 'All's well that ends well', and looked forward to going to the Prayer Meeting to give public thanks for what the Lord is doing on our behalf.

CHAPTER 32

The Waiting and A Reunion

5 December 2000 8.30am – I rang the Social Services Department to advise them of the situation and Gareth's Manager said that Gareth had gone home ill yesterday and didn't know if he would be at work today. However, she confirmed that there was no problem as someone else would speak to Mr Llewellyn in Gareth's absence. It's just for us to wait and see what happens next I suppose. Waiting... waiting... waiting... waiting. Meanwhile we picked Alwyn's mother up in the car and spent the afternoon at 'Young at Heart'. Dad said he enjoyed himself at the service at the Centre when I spoke to him on the phone this evening. I'm so glad that Dad still has the capacity at the moment to enjoy things, and I am resolved that, whatever happens in the future, I will do my best to ensure that he continues to engage in meaningful activities as far as he possibly can. I am realistic enough to know that Dad's condition is going to get worse, but until such a time is reached, let's help him all we can.

6 December 2000 Gareth rang from home to say that his Manager had told him of the latest developments. He said that he would like Dad to see the place where he was going to live and had arranged a viewing for tomorrow (Thursday). He said he would meet Alwyn and me at the Day Unit at 10.30am after Sian had explained to Dad what was going to happen. However, it was later suggested by Sian, that it would be better if Dad were told on Friday morning. This would avoid any unnecessary distress to Dad on Thursday night if he were to dwell on the matter of him having to move the next day. Sian said that past experience had shown that this was by far the best way to approach things and so I agreed to pick up Dad after lunch on Friday and meet Gareth at 2pm outside Seion.

7 December 2000 7.30am – I rang Dad to remind him, once again, that it was 'Day Centre Day' and he said, 'Why do the Government keep changing the clocks all the time Shirl? I've been down the shop but they're not open yet. No-one seems to want to keep to regular times these days. It was never like this when I was a boy. There's just no system with anyone from what I can see of it – it doesn't make sense! Anyway, what did you say, Shirl? Someone will come to pick me up for the Day Centre soon? Well if they don't come by nine o'clock – I'm off!' I reassured him that the driver would be along and told Dad that I'd ring this afternoon when he'd come back home.

Surely, the Lord does work in mysterious ways. This afternoon, after a concert at the Day Centre, one of the Carers brought someone over to sit next to Dad. In Dad's words it was 'my third sister who I hadn't seen for years. She was in the next Ward with eye trouble. She gave me a calendar which she'd made herself.' When I made enquiries, it turned out that the lady in question was my father's half-sister, Hazel, who was a permanent in-patient at Ysbyty Cwm Rhondda. I told Dad that, now we knew where Aunty Hazel was, we would be able to take him to visit her sometimes after all this time of being apart. He said that he would like that, so I've made a mental note of taking Dad to see her once things have settled down a bit with his circumstances.

The evening that followed was a long one. With so much to think about and so much to do the next day, I determined that the more time I spent in prayer the better prepared I would be spiritually and physically to deal with what was soon to take place. The promise is given in God's Word that 'They that wait upon the

Lord shall renew their strength, they shall mount up with wings as eagles; they shall run, and not be weary; and they shall walk, and not faint' (Isaiah 40:31).

CHAPTER 33

The Day Has Come

8 December 2000 After committing the day to the Lord in prayer, I began writing my list of 'Things To Do'. It looked something like this:-

1) 7.30am – Ring Dad (usual prompt for Day Centre)
2) Ring Sian to arrange time to pick up Dad
3) Ring Mr Llewellyn (Seion) to confirm time of arrival
4) Pick up Dad's clothes and personal belongings
5) Hand in completed forms to DSS
6) Lunch
7) Pick up Dad and deliver Christmas cards etc to Day Centre
8) Take Dad to his new home and settle him in
9) Visit Alwyn's mother
10) Visit Dad at our usual time of 6.30pm
11) Return home

Providentially, there were no 'hiccoughs' this morning with regard to Dad going to the Day Centre – everything went well. Thank You Lord! Sian said that she would explain to Dad that today was the day when he would be going to his new home and that Alwyn and I would be picking him up after lunch at 1.15pm. Once this time had been arranged, I rang Mr Llewellyn to advise him that we would be arriving at 2pm along with Mr Gareth Morris, Dad's Social Worker – so far – so good. Alwyn and I then left our home to journey to Dad's flat for what turned out to be the last but one time. On entering the flat, I felt as if all the memories of the time spent here with Mam and Dad had come to meet me. It was a strange sensation – one that will not easily be forgotten. However, I must not be distracted from the task in hand and the voice of practicality nudged me back into the present. I'd made another list of specific things that I needed to include for Dad's new home. There were the family photographs, Dad's miners' lamp he'd received on the occasion of his retirement (nearly twenty years ago), the Welsh doll that Alwyn's mother had made for my mother, the 'Mum and Dad' wall plaque with inscription, the 'World's Best Grandma and Grandpa' ornaments that the boys had presented so long ago . . .

The phone rang – it was Gareth. He said he wanted to find out how we were as he knew that today would be a difficult day for us and that, if we'd rather leave things until Sunday, then he'd arrange it. Apparently, Dad's room would not be ready until then, but there was still accommodation available today, but it would be on a sharing basis. Gareth said for us to think it over but after a quick prayer I said that as Dad is usually at his worst on the weekend it would be better if we went ahead as planned. This way, Dad would be having company over the weekend, albeit in new surroundings, rather than spending time in lonely confusion. It is true that you can be lonely in a crowd too, but in Dad's circumstances, I feel that the safety aspect has to come into view and so it was agreed – it has to be today – 2pm at Seion. My strong support throughout (though not physically, bless him!) made us yet another hot cup of tea and we sat on the settee – opposite 'the chair', Dad's chair. Enshrouded with coal dust from a bygone age, hugging to itself in the corner a cushion filled with 'hidden things' such as a rather grubby looking Tubigrip bandage, a rolled up writing pad, one of Mam's wigs and a spare cushion cover. I found myself closing the zip with a kind of holy reverence for it seemed to me that I was intruding on something very personal and private and I cried outwardly and apologized inwardly to Dad for such an intrusion. As I said before, whenever I asked Dad for an explanation of what had happened (such as the breakdown of the microwave cooker) his immediate response was 'It wasn't me! If I don't move from this chair!' Well, here we were and the chair was empty and Dad was about to embark upon another chapter in his life.

We arrived at the Day Centre car park at 1pm. Just enough time to offer one more prayer before meeting Dad. As I looked over the treetops, the Welsh hills seemed to be closer today somehow. Then I was reminded of the verse, 'I will lift up mine eyes unto the hills, from whence cometh my help. My help cometh from the Lord which made heaven and earth' (Psalm 121:1-2). Surely that was true of today as I know that, of my own strength, I could not go through this ordeal. If the Lord prayed, 'Not my will, but Thine be done', then I too must bow to the same principle in my life. Only the Lord can give me the courage to face what lies ahead. I understand, too, that Dad must be in pain as there are corridors of confusion running through his mind and I pray that the Lord will bring to his remembrance the times of long ago when he sat, as a child, under the ministry of the Gospel whilst at his mother's knee. I pray that these thoughts will bring him a measure of peace and that the God of grace will indeed give him comfort.

The car drew up at the entrance of the Day Centre and, taking a deep breath, I went inside. Dad was already dressed for the journey – his jacket, hat and overcoat were all on in the right order and he was looking very smart. However, that was his outward appearance – his inner being was not in such good condition. What was going on behind the scenes, I wonder? His blurry brown eyes portrayed a different picture. His stammering tongue wanted to say something but he just couldn't get the words out. Poor Dad. He was just a huddled frame of the man he once was – having to hold onto someone else for support whilst being accompanied to the sitting room to give his farewells to all the new friends he had made whilst attending the Day Centre. Hannah asked him if he'd like to give the ladies a goodbye kiss, but he declined the offer saying that he was too shy. Instead, he waved a shaky hand and wished them all the best before turning to me and said, 'OK love?' At this point, I was fighting back the floods of tears that were desperately trying to flow from behind eyes that were already red and swollen. I knew that this was not the time for my tears just yet, but for God's strength to be shown – I must be strong for Dad's sake. If I fall apart now, where would that leave Dad? No. There'll be plenty of time for tears later on – but in private! It feels the same now as in Mam's funeral – I had to be strong for Dad then and I have to be strong for Dad now. Hannah and I escorted Dad to the door and I ushered Dad into the front seat of the car. I sat next to Dad's suitcase on the back seat. From this position, I could place my hands on Dad's shoulders as he sat wiping a few tears from his eyes and cheeks. He tried to say something, but I couldn't quite make out the words. Then, as if he summoned all his powers of concentration, he said quite clearly, 'They tell me it's a nice place where I'm going, Shirl.' I began to tell him of the advantages of living somewhere where he didn't have to rummage around back lanes to find firewood, no more difficulty in trying to light the fire, no more hot coals on the carpet, no more 'waiting around the side-lines' as he used to say for someone to pick him up to take him to the Day Centre, he would be having his meals on a regular basis and someone was always on hand in case of any emergencies.

'Who will be paying for my rent, that's the thing though, Shirl? You sort my things out for me now don't you? What happens when I'm living somewhere else?' I reassured Dad that I would still be paying his rent from his pension as at present and that his other benefits would be going towards the cost of his upkeep as well. I told him not to worry as I had sorted everything out for him and that everything would be alright. He seemed to understand but his short-term memory is dreadful. So I determined that the best thing I could do, later on, would be to set out everything in a letter explaining what was happening (Please see Appendix 2) so that at least Dad would be able to read it for himself once the details were in writing and that, hopefully, he would be able to make a little sense out of it all. I can but hope and pray. We arrived fifteen minutes early and so Alwyn and I took advantage of this time and drove up to the lake which is situated about three quarters of a mile from Dad's new home. It was so peaceful. Again, the Welsh hillsides provided a source of beauty which is, in my view, unparalleled anywhere else on earth. I encouraged Dad with the thoughts of him being able to come up to this spot in the spring and summer months ahead with us and enjoy all the changing seasons – right on his new doorstep! He agreed that it was a wonderful sight and I began to quietly hum the tune 'How Great Thou Art' (One of Dad's favourite hymns).

However, we couldn't stay there all afternoon – there were things to do! We made our way back and as we arrived, Alwyn took charge of Dad's suitcase whilst I held firmly under Dad's arm and we all made our way up the path to the front door. Gareth greeted us outside and then rang the doorbell. 'Look up there, Dad!' I said pointing to the apex of the building. 'This used to be a church once upon a time, but now it has been converted into a home for the elderly, rather than be allowed to fall into disrepair.' 'That's a jolly good idea,' said Dad meaningfully and as we entered the building, he took off his cap and folded it away into his pocket with all due reverence and said, 'We must show respect for the House of the Lord, Shirl, mustn't we?' We were shown into Dad's temporary room which he was to share with Gwilym until Sunday. I admit it must have been bewildering to both Gwilym and Dad at first, but I pray that Dad will soon be able to make friends and that things will eventually settle down a bit. We were given a cup of tea and the first thing I did was to put Mam and Dad's framed photograph on the bedside cabinet so that Dad would have at least one thing familiar around him until we could put out everything we'd collected from his flat. I explained to Dad once again that he would be transferring to a room of his own downstairs on Sunday and then we would be able to come up and sort his things out properly. He said, 'That's alright, love, I'll be OK – you go off now and see to Alwyn's Mam.' I hugged and kissed him and said we'd be up to visit him later at our usual time of half past six. Whilst we were outside the building, we thanked Gareth for all his help throughout what had been a very difficult time for all of us as a family. 'If we don't see you before Christmas, all the best to you and your family, Gareth.' 'And the same to you,' Gareth replied as we all shook hands and went our separate ways.

When we got to Alwyn's mother's home, I just fell into her open arms and wept. Yes – we had another cup of tea as we related the morning's events. By this time, I was so exhausted as I hadn't slept much last night, and the day's events were beginning to take their toll. The settee in the front room looked so inviting and Alwyn's mother was ushering me lovingly towards it. I found myself now falling into the open arms of the settee and being covered up like a baby being put to bed for an afternoon nap. The last thing I heard was the room door sliding shut and the sound of the muffled voices of my husband and mother-in-law fading into the distance . . .

I awoke to the sound of tea cups rattling and Alwyn was gently shaking my shoulder, 'How are you feeling now, love? A bit better after a little sleep? Here's a cup of tea for you – we'll be getting ready soon to go up to see your father OK?' I roused myself and confessed that I did feel better after my little nap. Thank You Lord that You do give Your beloved sleep – even in the midst of difficult circumstances!

We found Dad to be rather unsettled which is what we expected if we were to be honest with ourselves. He said he thought he'd come home with us tonight if that was OK. I gently explained to him, yet again, that it was because of his medical condition that he needed to be living somewhere where someone could take care of him 24 hours a day and that Alwyn and I could not possibly undertake such a task. This was now to be his new home and, although it doesn't seem like it now, given time and patience by all concerned then it would eventually become home to him.

Before leaving, I reassured him that we would be up to see him again on Sunday and that Alwyn's mother would be up to visit too. He appeared to be a bit calmer when we left but I had a feeling that we were about to embark on a whole new series of episodes. However, that is another story.

Appendix 1

The following notes have been made as a result of attending the Day Unit at Ysbyty Cwm Rhondda, on Wednesday, 25 October at 6pm. The Lecture was given by Mrs Mair Jones of Newport. I trust that they will be helpful as well as informative.

Managing Difficult Behaviour
What is difficult behaviour? It could be any of the following:

Shouting, kicking, punching, spitting, biting, swearing, resisting, attention-seeking or moaning.

Why do we become difficult? Some of the likely reasons are suggested:

Organic illness, mental impairment, frustration, anger, epilepsy, learned behaviour, drugs, alcohol or FEAR.

Fear is one of the greatest contributing factors when difficult behaviour is the issue. When frightened, our body's self-defence mechanism goes into action and we do one of two things. Either we stay and fight or we run away – this has been termed 'Fight or Flight'. For example, how would your patient feel if you started to take their clothes off without explaining why? Very often you may be able to see the 'difficult' behaviour coming and the signs are shown in the patient's tone of voice, the content of the conversation, their facial expression and body language.

In order to offset this 'oncoming' behaviour and to diffuse what might become an upsetting situation, the following actions have been suggested:

Adopt an 'open' posture with your patient i.e. literally no pointing the finger, no hands on hips, no arm-folding, no threatening 'or else!' Your tone of voice should be calm – the same level and at normal volume. Shouting causes SHOUTING! Instead, try to convey trust, honesty, empathy (deeper than sympathy as you try and help the patient to feel that you want to help to understand how they feel) warmth, openness and genuineness.

Another aid to managing difficult behaviour is that of providing meaningful activities. If there is adequate stimulation, aggression decreases when the activity level is high. A chat, card game, dominoes etc can make a big difference. Just putting the patient to 'sit quietly and watch the TV' very often causes more harm as they get more withdrawn into their 'own world'.

Always treat your patient with respect and dignity. Above all, remember – you may not think your patient can understand you when he/she really can. Treat others as you would like to be treated yourself.

Appendix 2

23 December 2000

Dear Dad

This is probably the hardest letter that I have had to write – and the most painful. You see, as I've explained to you before, the Social Services Department have ruled that, in their assessment of things, you are no longer able to live alone as you are at risk both to yourself and others. Also, the Council are not prepared to rent you any of their properties for the same reason.

Therefore, the burden of responsibility has been placed on me to sort things out as far as the flat is concerned, whilst the Social Services Department's responsibility was to find you suitable alternative accommodation amongst other people with a similar medical condition to yourself.

So then, Dad, this is what has happened. Firstly, the only suitable accommodation in the local area so that Alwyn and I would still be able to visit you twice weekly as before, is where you are now – Seion Residential Home. However, should this prove to be unacceptable, the only other alternative would be somewhere much further away out of our area so that we couldn't come to visit you as regularly as we are now. If you remember, Dad, you always used to tell us when you were in your old flat and couldn't get the fire to light, '. . . and you wonder why I don't like it up here – I'm sorry I ever came to this hole!' Also, you had to go around the back lanes scrounging for firewood in all winds and weathers and come back home soaking wet and have to try and dry the wet sticks on top of the Parkray. Even though plans were made to convert the coal fire central heating to electric, the delays by the Council meant that, as every day went by, you were more at risk of death from hypothermia. However, it was deemed necessary to take action sooner rather than later and so it was decided that it was in your best interests medically to be moved into a safer environment.

The Council then had to take back possession of their flat and the task of sorting out your furniture and personal belongings passed to me. Dad, believe me, what a task that was! But under the circumstances, I was quite clear that it was a task I wanted to do on my own. Although I had offers of help, I simply wanted to be on my own when tackling such a job. So, where did I begin? First I notified the Area Housing Manager that all the furniture was to be taken to a re-cycling centre to be cleaned and given away to people in unfortunate circumstances. Secondly, any items of personal or sentimental value were sorted out and either brought to your new home or given to family members. I must confess, Dad, that I had a very hard time emotionally, dealing with these matters especially when I came across the cards in your wardrobe with your instructions of what you wanted me to do with them 'when our time comes' as you put it. Then finally, I had to take electricity meter readings and finalize the telephone bill and water rate details and then hand in all the keys to the Area Housing Manager last Monday.

So then, Dad, as you can appreciate, it was with a great sense of relief to me to know that you would now be in a safer, warmer and cleaner environment and living somewhere where you could be looked after 24 hours a day. Also, like you always told me, Dad, I was to take things easier and not to do so much because of my blood pressure problems. It was an answer to my prayers really when it was decided you could move into Seion, as another good thing about it was the fact that all your laundry needs would be taken care of by the staff at the home. At this point, Dad, I must re-emphasize – your new home is just that – it is a Residential Home, not a hospital, not an asylum, not a 'nut house', not a 'cave in the side of the mountain'. As in the case of the old flat, I've sorted out your cost of living at your new home and so there is no cause for any financial worry for you at all, OK Dad?'

So please, please Dad, for everyone's sake, try to come to terms with what is happening and indeed with what has happened, because although Seion is not your 'own home', if you remember you always said that after Mam died, 'this flat is not my own home – only a place for me to lay my head at night'.

I know it must be difficult and frustrating for you Dad, but believe me, it is equally hard for me too. I know that the Lord will look after us all, whatever comes our way as I've proved His loving-kindness over the many years that I have served Him. So Dad, let's look positively to the future and trust that together, as a family, we will learn to depend more upon the Lord in the year 2001 than we ever did before. With all my love, as always,

Shirley.

Useful Contacts

Rhondda Cynon Taff Carers' Support Project
CarersLine, Carers Pack and information for all carers in Rhondda Cynon Taff.
Freephone: 0808 100 1801
Freephone Minicom: 0808 100 1675
Email: Nigel. R. Billingham@rhondda-cynon-taff.gov.uk

Carers National Association Wales
River House
Ynysbridge Court
Gwaelod y Garth
Cardiff
CF15 9SS
Tel: 02920 811370
Fax: 02920 811575

Alzheimer's Disease Society Wales
4th Floor, Baltic House
Mount Stuart Square
Cardiff
CF10 5FH
Tel: 02920 431990
Fax: 02920 431999
Email: rows@alzheimers.org.uk

Dementia Careline
For carers of people with memory problems or Alzheimer's.
Tel: 02920 529848/9

Alpha
Reverend E. Banwell
14 Ffordd Llanbad
Gilfach Goch
CF39 8FL
Tel: 01443 674090